CALIFORNIA STATE UNI

This book is due on the last date stamped below.
Failure to return books on the date due will result in assessment
of overdue fees.

Neurologic Disorders in Women

Neurologic Disorders in Women

Edited by

Merit E. Cudkowicz, M.D.

Instructor in Neurology, Harvard Medical School, Boston; Assistant in
Neurology, Massachusetts General Hospital, Boston

Michael C. Irizarry, M.D.

Instructor in Neurology, Harvard Medical School, Boston; Assistant in
Neurology, Massachusetts General Hospital, Boston

With a Foreword by
Martin A. Samuels, M.D.
Professor of Neurology, Harvard Medical School, Boston; Neurologist-in-
Chief, Brigham and Women's Hospital, Boston

Butterworth–Heinemann
Boston   Oxford   Johannesburg   Melbourne   New Delhi   Singapore

Every effort has been made to ensure that the drug dosage schedules within this text are accurate and conform to standards accepted at time of publication. However, as treatment recommendations vary in the light of continuing research and clinical experience, the reader is advised to verify drug dosage schedules herein with information found on product information sheets. This is especially true in cases of new or infrequently used drugs.

∞ Recognizing the importance of preserving what has been written, Butterworth–Heinemann prints its books on acid-free paper whenever possible.

Library of Congress Cataloging-in-Publication Data
Neurologic disorders in women / [edited by] Merit E. Cudkowicz,
   Michael C. Irizarry ; foreword by Martin A. Samuels.
        p.   cm.
     Includes bibliographical references and index.
     ISBN 0-7506-9745-8
     1. Nervous system--Diseases. 2. Women--Diseases. I. Cudkowicz,
Merit E.   II. Irizarry, Michael C.
     [DNLM: 1. Nervous System Diseases. 2. Women's Health.   WL 140
     N4916 1997]
     RC346.N3837   1997
     616.8'082--dc21
     DNLM/DLC
     for Library of Congress   96-50469
                                                                   CIP

British Library Cataloguing-in-Publication Data
A catalogue record for this book is available from the British Library.

The publisher offers special discounts on bulk orders of this book.
For information, please contact:
Manager of Special Sales
Butterworth–Heinemann
313 Washington Street
Newton, MA 02158–1626
Tel: 617-928-2500
Fax: 617-928-2620

For information on all B–H medical publications available, contact our World Wide Web home page at: http://www.bh.com/med

10 9 8 7 6 5 4 3 2 1

Printed in the United States of America

To Mom
MEC

To Mom, Dad, Steven, and Nelson
MCI

For true Philosophers, aflame with love of truth and wisdom, never find themselves so sage or so full of wisdom or so abounding in perception but that they cede place to truth from whomsoever or whensoever it comes. Nor are they so narrowminded as to believe that our forebears have passed on to us any skill or knowledge so complete in all respects and perfect that nothing is left for the industry and diligence of others to accomplish.

—William Harvey, 1628

Contents

Contributing Authors

Tracy Batchelor, M.D.
Instructor in Neurology, Harvard Medical School, Boston; Assistant in Neurology, Massachusetts General Hospital, Boston

Merit E. Cudkowicz, M.D.
Instructor in Neurology, Harvard Medical School, Boston; Assistant in Neurology, Massachusetts General Hospital, Boston

F. Michael Cutrer, M.D.
Instructor in Neurology, Harvard Medical School, Boston; Assistant in Neurology, Massachusetts General Hospital, Boston

Mark W. Faragher, B.Med.Sc., M.B.B.S., F.R.A.C.P.
Clinical and Research Fellow in Neurology, Harvard Medical School and Massachusetts General Hospital, Boston

Teresa Gómez-Isla, M.D., Ph.D.
Clinical and Research Fellow in Neurology, Harvard Medical School and Massachusetts General Hospital, Boston

Bradley T. Hyman, M.D., Ph.D.
Associate Professor of Neurology, Harvard Medical School and Massachusetts General Hospital, Boston

Michael C. Irizarry, M.D.
Instructor in Neurology, Harvard Medical School, Boston; Assistant in Neurology, Massachusetts General Hospital, Boston

Michael Schwarzschild, M.D., Ph.D.
Instructor in Neurology, Harvard Medical School, Boston; Clinical and Research Fellow in Neurology, Massachusetts General Hospital, Boston

Alan Z. Segal, M.D.
Clinical Fellow in Neurology, Harvard Medical School, Boston; Resident Neurologist, Massachusetts General Hospital, Boston

Foreword

Neurologic problems comprise one of the largest groups of symptoms for which people seek medical attention and are a common reason for a subspecialty consultation. Many of these disorders have a gender bias. Knowing this fact often helps the physician to make the correct diagnosis and therefore to direct therapy appropriately.

Certain common neurologic problems, such as stroke and transient ischemic attack, have subgroups that are found predominantly or exclusively in women (e.g., pregnancy-related venous occlusions and hypercoagulable states due to the use of the oral contraceptives). Other disorders such as epilepsy may have unique manifestations in women because of the effect of estrogen and progesterone on brain receptors. Certain brain tumors are much more common in women (e.g., meningiomas), and others may be exclusive to the realm of women's neurology (e.g., breast cancer metastases). The female gender and, in particular, pregnancy may have dramatic effects on the course of certain neurologic disorders such as multiple sclerosis, which often improves during pregnancy, and migraine, which often worsens. Finally, a number of general medical conditions with frequent neurologic manifestations, such as systemic lupus erythematosus, are much more common in women.

In the distant past, issues related to women's health were clearly ignored. Even the field of obstetrics and gynecology (OB/GYN) was filled with male physicians. In recent years women have entered medicine in increasing numbers and with this welcome change has come an expansion of interest in women's health issues, beyond OB/GYN and into general internal medicine and family practice. The scientific medical literature began to note interesting and important gender differences in the biology of disease and its clinical manifestations. The discipline of epidemiology led the way, followed by physiology, biochemistry, anatomy, molecular biology, and genetics. Much is now known about gender differences in medical science, but it is difficult to find the information in practical, comprehensible sources.

Merit Cudkowicz and Michael Irizarry have done a marvelous job and performed a great service in compiling *Neurologic Disorders in Women*. Its clear and authoritative chapters are organized to be accessible to the practitioner. The concepts are up to date and well referenced, making the book a scholarly reference in addition to a practical manual. I have already referred to it in my practice and teaching rounds, and I expect it will become a standard reference for all who care for women with neurologic problems. As health care delivery changes, this resource will be needed by generalists, as well as the specialists with particular needs in this regard, such as neurologists, neurosurgeons, psychiatrists, and obstetricians and gynecologists.

In an era when most new medical books simply rehash old ideas or provide monographs on super-specialized areas, it is a pleasure to read a truly fresh work that successfully addresses a common and important issue.

MARTIN A. SAMUELS

Preface

In all fields of medicine, there is a growing interest in refining health care practices to provide optimum care for women. This interest stems from a concern that women's health issues have been neglected in the past. Important gender differences exist in the epidemiology, pathophysiology, clinical course, and treatment of many neurologic diseases. Our goal in characterizing the features of neurologic diseases unique to women is to provide a resource to clinicians and to highlight areas that require further clinical and basic research.

This book is organized in nine chapters emphasizing the clinical aspects of neurologic diseases in women, including speculation on the neuroscientific basis for gender differences, particularly the role of female steroid hormones. Several disorders, including migraine, multiple sclerosis, meningiomas and pituitary adenomas, Alzheimer's disease, and antiphospholipid antibody syndrome, occur more commonly in women. Hormonal effects, particularly those of estrogen, have been implicated in influencing the clinical course of epilepsy, migraine, stroke, meningiomas, and even Alzheimer's disease. Many disorders that occur in young women—such as epilepsy, migraine, and multiple sclerosis—raise important issues regarding reproductive endocrine function, contraception, sexuality, and pregnancy.

We thank the many collaborators who have contributed to this review of the current knowledge of neurologic disorders in women.

MERIT E. CUDKOWICZ
MICHAEL C. IRIZARRY

Neurologic Disorders
in Women

CHAPTER 1

Epilepsy

Michael C. Irizarry

The incidence of epilepsy is slightly greater in males than in females; however, many medical issues are specific to the female with epilepsy. This chapter reviews the interactions of epilepsy with female sex hormones, menarche, menstruation, menopause, reproductive endocrine function, and pregnancy.

Epidemiology

Most recent epidemiologic studies report an increased incidence of epilepsy in males compared to females. The overall incidence of epilepsy in the American population (based on population-based studies from Rochester, Minnesota [1]) is greater in males (49 per 100,000 person-years) than in females (41 per 100,000 person-years). The corresponding cumulative incidence rates through age 74 are 3.4% in males and 2.8% in females. The gender difference in incidence rates is most pronounced in the oldest age groups; during the first 5 years of life, females have a slightly higher incidence, especially of generalized seizures. The increased incidence in males versus females is found in partial (28 versus 24 per 100,000 person-years), generalized (20 versus 15 per 100,000 person-years), idiopathic (31 versus 27 per 100,000 person-years), and remote symptomatic (18 versus 14 per 100,000 person-years) epilepsy. Among individual seizure types, the incidence for each category of partial epilepsy (simple, complex, and secondarily generalized) and for generalized tonic-clonic seizures is greater in males; the incidence is equal between genders for myoclonic seizures (1 per 100,000 person-years); and the incidence of absence seizures is higher in females (3 versus 2 per 100,000 person-years in males) [1]. Among the epilepsy syndromes, childhood absence and epilepsy with photosensitivity are preponderant in females; epilepsy is also associated with Rett syndrome and Aicardi's syndrome, both of which occur exclusively in females [2].

The incidence of first unprovoked seizure is also greater in males than in females (68 versus 56 per 100,000 person-years, cumulative incidence 4.7% versus 3.7%) [1]; however, there is no significant gender difference in the 40–46% risk of recurrence within 2 years [3–5].

The rate of remission after discontinuation of medication is related more to etiology, electroencephalographic (EEG) pattern, seizure type, epilepsy syndrome, and duration of seizure-free interval than to the gender of the patient [6].

Hormones and Epilepsy

The complex relationship between hormones, seizures, and anticonvulsants is clinically relevant to pregnancy, catamenial seizures, and reproductive endocrine function in women with epilepsy. The major steroid hormones estrogen and progesterone have opposing effects in animal models of seizures and in human studies. In animal seizure models, estrogen is proconvulsant, lowering maximal electroshock seizure and kindling thresholds [7] and eliciting spike generation with direct application to cortex [8]. Intravenous (IV) estrogens increased spike frequency in 11 of 16 females with epilepsy, producing grand mal seizures in four [9]. Proposed mechanisms for these effects include decreased gamma-aminobutyric acid (GABA) inhibition through the steroid recognition site on the GABA-A receptor complex, and possible regulation of glutamate receptors. Progesterone increases seizure threshold in maximal electroshock, phenylenetetrazol, and kindling models [8, 10, 11]. IV progesterone in the first week of the menstrual cycle significantly reduced spike frequency in four of seven women with distinct temporal lobe EEG foci [12]. Progesterone also acts through a putative steroid-binding site on the GABA-A receptor complex [13, 14]. In the rat, progesterone receptor binding is diffuse in the cortex, while estrogen receptor binding is concentrated in the preoptic area, hypothalamic region, and amygdala [15]. However, the anticonvulsant potency of synthetic progestins does not correlate with hormonal potency [11].

Menarche

Seizure patterns in women may change during menarche, menopause, the menstrual cycle, and pregnancy. Although the onset of puberty is associated with remission of childhood absence epilepsy and benign rolandic epilepsy, puberty does not significantly affect most seizure disorders [10]. In a study of 115 girls with established epilepsy, the course remained unchanged in 33%, seizure frequency increased or a new type of seizure occurred in 44%, and seizure frequency decreased or ceased in 22%. Individuals who have generalized tonic-clonic seizures, complex partial seizures, earlier onset or known etiology of seizure disorder, neurologic or psychological abnormalities on examination, abnormal EEG, and later onset of menarche are at risk for increased seizure activity during puberty [16, 17]. Other studies have shown a decrease in complex partial seizures with puberty [18, 19]. Most recent studies conclude that children with epilepsy experience a normal puberty [20].

Menopause

During menopause, improvement of seizure disorders has been associated with a late age of onset of menopause, a catamenial component, later onset of the seizure disorder, or infrequent seizures. Worsening of seizure disorders has been associated with an earlier onset of menopause, frequent generalized tonic-clonic seizures, and complex partial seizures [10, 17].

Catamenial Epilepsy

Catamenial epilepsy refers to a seizure disorder with periodic exacerbations in the menstrual or immediate premenstrual period. The exact incidence in females with epilepsy is unclear. Studies report increases in seizures several days before or during menses in 10–72% of females with epilepsy [21, 22]. Methodologic difficulties such as inexact documentation, cyclic seizures unrelated to menses, definition of the catamenial period, seizure types and severity, medications, follow-up, and anovulatory cycles contribute to the disparity [21]. The importance of good documentation of seizure occurrence was illustrated by a study of 120 menstrual cycles in 40 women with refractory epilepsy [23]. Although 78% of women believed that most seizures occurred near the time of or were exacerbated by menstruation, seizure diaries revealed that only 12.5% satisfied the study's definition of catamenial epilepsy, which specified that 75% of seizures occur either 4 days before or 6 days after the onset of menstruation. There is no correlation between the risk of catamenial exacerbation and the specific seizure type or seizure severity [21]. In addition to perimenstrual exacerbations, some studies have noted increases in seizure frequency during the preovulatory period [24] and in midcycle [25].

The role of pituitary and ovarian hormones in epilepsy and catamenial epilepsy has been investigated. Backstrom [24] measured estrogen and progesterone levels during six ovulatory cycles in five patients with uncontrolled secondarily generalized seizures. Seizure frequency was positively correlated with the estrogen/progesterone ratio; secondarily generalized seizures increased during menstruation (after the rapid decrease in plasma progesterone) and at the time of increasing preovulatory estrogen. There was no relationship between hormonal parameters and partial seizures. Seizure frequency of both partial and generalized seizures was positively correlated with estrogen level in a study of three anovulatory cycles in three patients [24]. There was no consistent covariation between hormone levels and anticonvulsant drug total levels [26]. An impairment of absolute or relative progesterone secretion is suggested by a study of 10 women with catamenial epilepsy that found a reduced progesterone/estrogen ratio compared to normal controls; however, this ratio was not significantly different from women without catamenial exacerbation of epilepsy. No difference was found in baseline luteinizing hormone (LH), follicle-stimulating hormone (FSH), and prolactin (PRL) levels; LH and FSH secretory response to gonadotropin-releasing hormone (GnRH); PRL response to thyrotropin-releasing hormone (TRH); or cyclic estrogen levels [27, 28]. Rosciszewska found increased excretion of urinary metabolites of estrogen and progesterone in women with epilepsy compared to controls, with inverse correlation between seizure frequency and progesterone metabolites. Patients with catamenial seizures had greater cycle variation in phenytoin (Dilantin) levels, but not in phenobarbital levels [29]. It is unclear from these data if absolute hormone levels, estrogen/progesterone ratios, or sensitivity to hormonal changes differs significantly in women with catamenial epilepsy as compared to women without catamenial exacerbation of seizures.

Treatments for catamenial epilepsy include perimenstrual supplementation of anticonvulsants, intermittent diuretics, and hormones. Drug levels can be measured perimenstrually, with supplementation of the patient's usual anticonvulsant medication if necessary [30]. Oral acetazolamide, 250–750 mg per day, started 10 days before anticipated menses and continued throughout menstruation, has been suggested as an adjunctive therapy [30, 31]. Hormonal interventions have been evaluated in several small studies. In 12 patients with complex partial seizures and reproductive endocrine disorders, the estrogen analogue clomiphene citrate reduced overall seizure frequency by 87% [32]. Vaginal progesterone suppositories of 50–400 mg given every 12 hours in the latter half of the menstrual cycle reduced seizures in eight women by 68% [33], and progesterone lozenges at 200 mg three times a day in the latter half of the menstrual cycle reduced seizures in 25 women by 55% [34]. Oral medroxyprogesterone acetate, 10 mg two to four times daily, or intramuscular (IM) depot medroxyprogesterone, 120–150 mg every 6–12 weeks, reduced seizure frequency in seven of 14 females with intractable epilepsy by an average of 52% [35]. In 10 premenopausal women with catamenial seizures, triptorelin, a GnRH analogue, eliminated seizures in three, and reduced seizures by up to 50% in four others [36]. The benzodiazepine clobazam, 20–30 mg orally for a 10-day perimenstrual period, was effective supplementation in 14 of 18 patients with catamenial epilepsy [37, 38].

Reproductive Endocrine Function

While normal hormonal changes during the menstrual cycle may affect seizure frequency, epilepsy itself may influence hormonal balance, as women with epilepsy have an increased incidence of sexual dysfunction and reproductive endocrine dysfunction. Hyposexuality with disinterest and lack of libido is frequently described in patients of both sexes with epilepsy, particularly in those with temporal lobe epilepsy (TLE) [11]. Two-thirds of patients undergoing temporal lobectomy for epilepsy had sexual disturbances, primarily hyposexuality, that sometimes improved with better seizure control [39]. Disorders in sexual arousal and sexual desire have been characterized in a study of nine females with TLE [40]. The females with TLE described significantly fewer sexual experiences, less arousal, and more anxiety about imagined sexual activities compared to females without epilepsy as measured by the Sexual Behavior Inventory, Sexual Arousability Inventory, and Sexual Anxiety Inventory. Physiologically, the females with TLE had diminished genital blood flow responses to sexually explicit stimuli, despite normal subjective ratings of arousal.

Menstrual and reproductive endocrine dysfunction is frequent in both TLE and primary generalized epilepsy (PGE). In a study of 50 women with TLE, 56% had menstrual dysfunction and 38% had reproductive endocrine disorders. Menstrual dysfunction included amenorrhea in 16% of the total, oligomenorrhea in 20%, and abnormal menstrual cycle interval in 20%. Reproductive endocrine disorders included polycystic ovarian syndrome (PCO) in 20% of the group, hypothalamic hypogonadism (HH) in 12%, premature menopause (PM) in 4%, and hyperprolactinemia (HP) in 2%. The estimated frequency of these disorders in the general population is PCO 5%, HH 1.5%, PM 1%, and HP 1%. There was no significant relationship between menstrual disorders and medication, although PCO was more common among untreated women (13.5% of treated versus 30% of untreated) and HH was more common in treated women (17% of treated versus 5% of untreated) [41]. Other studies have found a high prevalence (61–64%) of PCO or hyperandrogenism with long-term valproate therapy [42, 43]. In women with reproductive endocrine disorders and lateralized temporal discharges, PCO has been associated with left-sided foci in over 90% and HH with right temporal foci in over 85% [41, 44].

Menstrual dysfunction and reproductive endocrine disorders have also been described in women with PGE. A study of 20 women with PGE found menstrual dysfunction in 30% (5% amenorrhea, 20% oligomenorrhea, 5% polymenorrhea) and reproductive endocrine disorders in 25% (15% PCO, 10% HH) [45]. Disordered ovulatory function, however, may be more common in TLE than in PGE. Ovulatory function was assessed in 20 cycles in seven women with PGE, 45 cycles in 17 women with TLE, and 35 cycles in 12 controls. Anovulation as determined by basal temperatures and serum progesterone level at day 21 of the menstrual cycle was significantly more common in women with TLE (seven of 45 cycles in six of 12 subjects) compared to women with PGE (no anovulatory cycles) and controls (one anovulatory cycle), independent of seizure activity, although possibly associated with polytherapy [46].

Dysregulation of opposing amygdala corticobasal nucleus and basolateral nucleus control over hypothalamic GnRH and dopamine systems has been postulated as a mechanism for the association of TLE with reproductive endocrine and menstrual disorders [41]. Impaired LH response to GnRH, abnormal early follicular LH levels, and altered pulse frequency of LH have been described in TLE [45, 47, 48], as well as a possible anticonvulsant-related decreased LH pulse frequency [48]. Other hormonal effects of anticonvulsant medication have been described. Carbamazepine treatment alters sex hormone balance, with decreased dehydroepiandrosterone sulfate (DHEA-S) level and free-androgen index, increased level of steroid hormone–binding globulin, and short-term decrease in LH and gonadotropin responsiveness to GnRH [49, 50]. Phenytoin also decreases DHEA-S [51]. Long-term valproate use has been associated with increased serum testosterone and increased DHEA-S [43].

Given these data, menstrual history should be assessed in all women with epilepsy. Some neurologists have recommended documenting basal body temperature, menses onset, and seizure occurrence. Follicular phase and luteal phase levels of LH, FSH, PRL, free and total testosterone, estradiol, and progesterone may identify specific patterns of neuroendocrine dysfunction amenable to hormonal therapy [30].

Cosmetic Effects of Anticonvulsants

Anticonvulsant-induced hormonal changes may be responsible for some of the cosmetic side effects of anticonvulsant medications. The strongest association is weight gain during valproate therapy, which occurs in 50% of patients and has been correlated with hyperinsulinism, hyperandrogenism, and PCO [43]. Other cosmetic side effects occur in both sexes and have an unclear hormonal association. Phenytoin, possibly in combination with phenobarbital, can cause coarsening of facial features, hirsutism, and gingival hyperplasia. Alopecia has been described with valproate, hair thinning with carbamazepine, weight gain with vigabatrin, and weight loss with felbamate [52, 53].

Oral Contraceptives

Contraceptive counseling is an important aspect in the care of premenopausal women with epilepsy, given the increased risk of complications of pregnancy as well as the teratogenic effects of anticonvulsant medications. Despite the putative epileptogenic effect of estrogen, oral contraceptives (OCPs) do not exacerbate seizure disorders [8, 54, 55]. OCP efficacy, however, is reduced as much as fourfold by hepatic enzyme–inducing anticonvulsant medications [56]. There have been at least 50 cases of OCP failures in association with anticonvulsant therapy documented in the literature [57]. Between 1974 and 1984, 43 cases of OCP failure associated with anticonvulsant medications were reported in the United Kingdom; the number of patients on each anticonvulsant were: phenytoin, 25; phenobarbital, 20; carbamazepine, six; primidone, seven; ethosuximide, four; and valproate, one (the latter two medications always used in polytherapy) [58]. In a retrospective analysis of females with epilepsy taking OCPs, three pregnancies occurred over 955 months in 41 women treated with anticonvulsants, compared to no pregnancies over 1,450 months in 41 untreated women, worsening the use effectiveness of OCPs from 0.7 pregnancies per 100 woman years to 3.1, a failure rate comparable to that of barrier methods of contraception [56]. Breakthrough bleeding occurred in 60–76% of women on standard OCPs taking carbamazepine, phenytoin, and phenobarbital, compared to 6% on valproate and none on benzodiazepines [57].

The primary cause of OCP failure is induction of microsomal enzymes by the anticonvulsants phenytoin, phenobarbital, carbamazepine, and primidone, resulting in insufficient synthetic steroid concentration to block ovulation [11]. Pharmacokinetic studies measuring synthetic hormone levels in four patients before and after receiving phenobarbital demonstrated a reduction of greater than 50% in ethinyl estradiol levels in two patients, without a change in progestin levels [59]. Both ethinyl estradiol and levonorgestrel levels decreased an average of 50% in six females taking phenytoin and four taking carbamazepine [60]. Benzodiazepines, ethosuximide, vigabatrin, lamotrigine, and gabapentin are not believed to alter OCP effectiveness since these drugs are negligibly bound to serum proteins and have no microsomal enzyme–inducing effect [61]. In studies specifically addressing this issue, lamotrigine did not significantly reduce ethinyl estradiol and levonorgestrel levels in 12 healthy female volunteers receiving a combined OCP [62]. Gabapentin also did not significantly affect norethindrone or ethinyl estradiol pharmacokinetics in 13 healthy female subjects [63]. Valproate, which inhibits microsomal enzymes, actually increased the peak concentration of ethinyl estradiol [64]. A similar effect could be postulated for felbamate, which also inhibits the hepatic microsomal enzyme system.

Although some have recommended other forms of birth control (such as intrauterine devices and barrier methods) for women with epilepsy based on these drug interactions [65], most physicians do not regard the combination OCP as contraindicated and, in fact, recommend OCPs based on the high efficacy in this high-risk group [8]. The usual equivalent dose of 30 µg estrogen is insufficient to suppress ovulation in women taking microsomal enzyme–inducing anticonvulsant medications; a combined OCP medication containing at least 50 µg estrogen is required [66]. Breakthrough bleeding is an unreliable indicator of contraceptive failure, and assessing suppression of luteal phase progesterone by measuring blood progesterone concentration on day 21 of the first cycle (if the OCP was started on days 1–3) or second cycle (if the OCP was started on days 3–5) may be more reliable [66]. The estrogen dose can be increased to 60 µg, 80 µg, or up to 100 µg using combinations of OCP containing 30 µg and 50 µg estrogen until ovulation has been suppressed [66, 67]. IM depot medroxyprogesterone acetate, 150 mg, every three months is also an alternative means of contraception; other long-acting sustained-release progestins such as levonorgestrel may not be as effective [8]. At least twice the dose of the progestin-only pill may be required [66]. Since the metabolites of estrogen and progesterone are toxicologically inactive, the increased doses of hormones required to suppress ovulation in women taking enzyme-inducing anticonvulsants should not result in any increase in side effects compared to the 30 µg dose of estrogen in women not taking anticonvulsants [68].

Pregnancy

Every female with epilepsy should be aware of the risks and possible complications of pregnancy related both to medications and the seizure disorder itself, although over 90% of pregnancies in this population deliver healthy babies [69]. A prospective study of approximately 45,000 pregnant women determined that 4.5 per 1,000 pregnant women had experienced seizures in the previous 5 years, and that 4.4 per 1,000 women experienced a noneclamptic seizure during pregnancy [70]. Reviews of prospective studies of pregnancy in women with epilepsy found that 17–34% experienced an increase in seizure frequency, 13–25% a decrease, and 50–83% no change [11, 69]. Increased seizure frequency does not correlate with age, seizure type, anticonvulsant medication, or prior pregnancy [69]. The major factors involved in increased seizure frequency are noncompliance with medications and sleep deprivation [71], although hormonal changes (increased estrogen or beta-human chorionic gonadotropin) [72], physiologic changes (increased weight, fluid and sodium retention, respiratory alkalosis, hypomagnesemia), altered anticonvulsant pharmacokinetics, stress, and poor seizure control before conception may play a role [69, 73]. In a study of 51 pregnancies, the total serum levels of carbamazepine, phenytoin, phenobarbital, and valproate decreased by 42%, 56%, 55%, and 39%, respectively, during the course of the pregnancy; free levels of carbamazepine, phenytoin, and phenobarbital decreased to a lesser extent (28%, 31%, and 50%, respectively), while that of valproate increased by 25% [74]. For phenytoin and phenobarbital, the greatest decline was in the first trimester, while that of carbamazepine was in the third trimester [74]. Recommendations for drug monitoring during pregnancy have included drawing a preconception baseline total and free level and routine total levels every two months [69]. Monthly free levels have been suggested for patients with poorly controlled seizures, patients with increased seizure frequency, or patients with over 50% decline in total levels [69]. Changes in anticonvulsant drug dosages are dictated primarily by the clinical state of the patient rather than the drug levels. Dosages may need to be reduced postpartum to prepregnancy levels to avoid toxicity [75].

Status epilepticus during pregnancy occurs in less than 1% of women with epilepsy and may be associated with increased maternal or fetal mortality. Treatment of status epilepticus not associated with eclampsia is the same as for the nonpregnant patient, with the addition of the use of a fetal heart monitor [72]. IV benzodiazepines have been recommended for noneclamptic seizures, which occur in 1–2% of women with epilepsy during labor and in 1–2% during the 24 hours after delivery [76].

Women with epilepsy appear to be at an increased risk for obstetric complications and poor pregnancy outcome. Fertility itself is reduced to 69–85% of that expected [77, 78]. There is a 1.5- to 4.0-fold increase in obstetric complications including vaginal bleeding (in 7–10%), preeclampsia, anemia, hyperemesis gravidarum, maternal herpes, placenta previa, and placental abruption; these are associated with a two- to fourfold increase in obstetric interventions including second- or third-trimester amniocentesis, induced labor, and cesarean section [69, 79]. Adverse pregnancy outcomes such as prematurity (4–11%), low birth weight (7–10%), low Apgar score, stillbirth, and perinatal and neonatal death are increased twofold. Vitamin K deficiency, feeding difficulties, developmental delay, and anticonvulsant drug withdrawal can complicate the postnatal period in the infant [69, 80]. Because of the high mortality rate (25–33%) from internal hemorrhage due to competitive inhibition of transplacental transport of vitamin K by anticonvulsant medications [80], all infants of mothers taking these medications should receive 1 mg of IM vitamin K at birth [75]. In addition, 10–20 mg daily of oral vitamin K for pregnant mothers in the last 2–4 weeks of pregnancy is recommended [66, 69].

The association of fetal malformations with epilepsy and anticonvulsant medications has been evaluated in many studies. Yerby reviewed 39 studies of malformation rates in children of mothers with and without epilepsy from 1956 to 1992 and concluded that infants of mothers with epilepsy have a two- to threefold increase in the rate of congenital malformations. The malformation rate for these children averaged 4–8% (with a range of 2.3–18.6%), compared to 2–3% for the general population [80]. Medications have been implicated as the major risk factor for congenital malformations in offspring of mothers with epilepsy, as higher rates have been observed in treated groups than in untreated groups, with higher serum anticonvulsant concentrations, and with polytherapy. It is not clear if seizures during pregnancy affect the risk of congenital malformations

[80]. Estimates of the incidence of congenital malformations when the mother takes no, one, two, three, or four anticonvulsant drugs are 2%, 3%, 5.5%, 11%, and 23%, respectively [61]. Malformations linked to phenobarbital, primidone, and phenytoin include cleft lip and palate (1.8% for phenytoin compared to 0.7% in the general population [66]), congenital heart disease (atrial septal defect, ventricular septal defect), skeletal abnormalities, and intestinal atresia. An increased risk of spina bifida aperta has been associated with valproate (1–2%) and carbamazepine (0.5–1.0%) over phenobarbital and phenytoin (0.3–0.4%) [52, 81]. In addition, specific fetal anticonvulsant drug syndromes for trimethadione, phenytoin, primidone, phenobarbital, valproate, and carbamazepine have been described, consisting of varying combinations of midfacial dysmorphism, distal digital hypoplasia, intrauterine growth retardation, developmental delay, and heart defects [80]. Prospective studies have suggested that the incidence of these syndromes is quite low (except for fetal trimethadione syndrome, which occurs in up to 87%; trimethadione is contraindicated in pregnancy), and that minor dysmorphic features may resolve during childhood [76, 80, 81]. Mechanisms suggested for anticonvulsant teratogenesis include toxic effects of free radical or arene epoxide metabolites of aromatic anticonvulsants, and effects on folate metabolism [80]. The teratogenicity of the newer anticonvulsant medications is still not known, although normal deliveries have been reported in women receiving gabapentin and felbamate [82]. Given these data, recommendations have been made to evaluate the need for medication in young women with epilepsy, and to treat with the lowest dose and fewest medications necessary to control seizures, preferably using monotherapy. Amniotic fluid or serum analysis of alpha-fetoprotein at 16 weeks of pregnancy and ultrasonography at 18–19 weeks in women taking valproate or carbamazepine can detect neural tube defects; ultrasonography at 20–24 weeks has been suggested to evaluate for heart malformations and facial clefts in women taking other anticonvulsants [76]. A diet rich in folate or folate supplements (0.4–1.0 mg per day) has been recommended before conception [66]. High doses of folate (2–4 mg per day) are suggested if there is a family history of neural tube defects [69].

Evaluation and treatment of seizures in a pregnant woman are similar to that of other seizure patients. A seizure disorder may first become manifest during pregnancy. One-fourth of these women will have gestational epilepsy, with seizures only during pregnancy. Only one-third will experience a recurrence of seizures during subsequent pregnancies [83]. Women who are past 20 weeks of gestation need to be evaluated for eclampsia with associated hypertension, proteinuria, and edema, which warrants vigorous intervention [72]. Eclampsia complicates one in 2,000 deliveries, and recent studies support the use of magnesium sulfate as the therapeutic agent of choice for prevention and treatment of eclamptic seizures [84]. In a prospective trial of 2,138 women with hypertension in pregnancy (systolic blood pressure >140 mm Hg and diastolic blood pressure >90 mm Hg), 10 of 1,089 treated with therapeutic blood levels of phenytoin progressed to eclamptic seizures, compared to none of 1,049 treated with a protocol of IM or IV magnesium sulfate. Intrapartum maternal outcomes and infant outcomes did not significantly differ among the two groups, although most of the 10 women with eclamptic seizures had peripartum complications including cesarean section and low–birth weight infants [85]. The Eclampsia Trial Collaborative Group compared IV or IM magnesium sulfate to IV diazepam or IV phenytoin for treatment of established eclamptic seizure. Magnesium sulfate reduced recurrent convulsions by 52% compared with diazepam and 67% compared with phenytoin. Maternal and fetal outcomes also favored magnesium sulfate treatment [86]. Protocols for magnesium sulfate administration in these trials were a 10-g IM loading dose in divided doses in each buttock followed by 5 g IM every 4 hours, or a 4-g IV loading dose followed by 1 g per hour by IV. Maintenance doses were given provided patellar reflexes were present, respirations exceeded 12 per minute, and urine output was maintained at over 25 ml per hour [85, 86]. Additional therapeutic measures include hydralazine, 5–10 mg IV every 15–20 minutes, for diastolic blood pressure over 110 mm Hg and delivery of the baby when feasible [72].

In the puerperium, considerations include breast-feeding and maternal seizures. All anticonvulsants are secreted into the breast milk, with a breast-milk concentration relative to maternal serum concentration of 2–5% for valproate; 18–45% for phenytoin, phenobarbital, and carbamazepine; 60–70% for primidone; and 90% for ethosuximide [83, 87]. Breast-feeding may be contraindicated in women taking medications such as phenobarbital and primidone if there is associated irritability, poor feeding, or slow weight gain in the infant [66]. Mothers should take precautions to protect the infant in the event of a maternal seizure, such as feeding and changing the baby on the floor and supervision while bathing the infant [66, 69].

Conclusion

Physicians need to counsel women with epilepsy regarding the reciprocal effects of seizures and the menstrual cycle, pregnancy, anticonvulsant medications, and OCPs. Vigilance for complicating reproductive endocrine disorders and monitoring during pregnancy are essential.

References

1. Hauser WA. Incidence of epilepsy and unprovoked seizures in Rochester, Minnesota: 1935–1984. Epilepsia 1993;34:453.
2. Wallace SJ. Epileptic Syndromes of Childhood and Adolescence. In MR Trimble (ed), Women and Epilepsy. New York: Wiley, 1991;107.

3. Hauser WA. Seizure recurrence after a first unprovoked seizure. N Engl J Med 1982;307:522.
4. Hopkins A, Garman A, Clarke C. The first seizure in adult life: value of clinical features, electroencephalography, and computed tomographic scanning in prediction of seizure recurrence. Lancet 1988;1:721.
5. van Donselaar CA, Geerts AT, Schimsheimer R. Idiopathic first seizure in adult life: who should be treated? BMJ 1991;302:620.
6. Shinnar S, Berg AT. Withdrawal of antiepileptic drugs. Curr Opin Neurol 1995;8:103.
7. Hom AC, Buterbaugh GG. Estrogen alters the acquisition of seizures kindled by repeated amygdala stimulation or pentylenetetrazol administration in ovariectomized female rats. Epilepsia 1986;27:103.
8. Mattson RH, Rebar RW. Contraceptive methods for women with neurologic disorders. Am J Obstet Gynecol 1993;168:2027.
9. Logothetis J, Harner R, Morrel F, et al. The role of estrogens in catamenial exacerbation of epilepsy. Neurology 1959;9:352.
10. Morrell MJ. Hormones and epilepsy through the lifetime. Epilepsia 1992;33(Suppl 4):S49.
11. Mattson RH, Cramer JA. Epilepsy, sex hormones, and antiepileptic drugs. Epilepsia 1985;26(Suppl 1):S40.
12. Backstrom T, Zetterlund B, Blom S, et al. Effects of intravenous progesterone infusions on the epileptic discharge frequency in women with partial epilepsy. Acta Neurol Scand 1984;69:240.
13. Belelli D, Bolger MB, Gee KW. Anticonvulsant profile of the progesterone metabolite 5α-pregnan-3α-ol-20-one. Eur J Pharmacol 1989;166:325.
14. Gee KW, Bolger MB, Brinton RE, et al. Steroid modulation of the chloride ionophore in rat brain: structure-activity requirements, regional dependence and mechanism of action. J Pharmacol Exp Therap 1988;246:803.
15. Maggi A, Perez J. Role of female gonadal hormones in the CNS: clinical and experimental aspects. Life Sci 1985;37:893.
16. Rosciszewska D. Epilepsy and Menstruation. In A Hopkins (ed), Epilepsy. London: Chapman & Hall Medical, 1987;373.
17. Kurtz Z. Sex Differences in Epilepsy: Epidemiological Aspects. In MR Trimble (ed), Women and Epilepsy. New York: Wiley, 1991;47.
18. Niijima S, Wallace SJ. Effects of puberty on seizure frequency. Dev Med Child Neurol 1989;31:174.
19. Diamantopoulos N, Crumrine P. The effect of puberty on the course of epilepsy. Arch Neurol 1986;43:873.
20. Macardle BM, McGowen ME, Greene SA, et al. Anticonvulsant drugs, growth, and development. Arch Dis Child 1987;62:615.
21. Newmark ME, Penry JK. Catamenial epilepsy: a review. Epilepsia 1980;21:281.
22. Crawford P. Catamenial Seizures. In MR Trimble (ed), Women and Epilepsy. New York: Wiley, 1991;159.
23. Duncan S, Read CL, Brodie MJ. How common is catamenial epilepsy? Epilepsia 1993;34:827.

24. Backstrom T. Epileptic seizures in women related to plasma estrogen and progesterone during the menstrual cycle. Acta Neurol Scand 1976;54:321.
25. Herkes GK, Eadie MJ, Sharbrough F, et al. Patterns of seizure occurrence in catamenial epilepsy. Epilepsy Res 1993;15:47.
26. Backstrom T, Jorpes P. Serum phenytoin, phenobarbital, carbamazepine, albumin, and plasma estradiol, progesterone concentrations during the menstrual cycle in women with epilepsy. Acta Neurol Scand 1979;59:63.
27. Murri L, Bonuccelli U, Melis GB. Neuroendocrine evaluation in catamenial epilepsy. Funct Neurol 1986;1:399.
28. Bonuccelli U, Melis GB, Paoletti AM, et al. Unbalanced progesterone and estradiol secretion in catamenial epilepsy. Epilepsy Res 1989;3:100.
29. Rosciszewska D, Buntner B, Guz I, et al. Ovarian hormones, anticonvulsant drugs, and seizures during the menstrual cycle in women with epilepsy. J Neurol Neurosurg Psychiatr 1986;49:47.
30. Schachter SC. Neuroendocrine aspects of epilepsy. Neurol Clin 1994;12:31.
31. Engle J. Seizures and Epilepsy. In F Plum (ed), Contemporary Neurology Series. Philadelphia: FA Davis, 1989;536.
32. Herzog AG. Clomiphene therapy in epileptic women with menstrual disorders. Neurology 1988;38:432.
33. Herzog AG. Intermittent progesterone therapy and frequency of complex partial seizures in women with menstrual disorders. Neurology 1986;36:1607.
34. Herzog AG. Progesterone therapy in women with complex partial and secondarily generalized seizures. Neurology 1995;45:1660.
35. Mattson RH, Cramer JA, Caldwell BV, et al. Treatment of seizures with medroxyprogesterone acetate: preliminary report. Neurology 1984;34:1255.
36. Bauer J, Wildt L, Flugel D, et al. The effect of a synthetic GnRH analogue on catamenial epilepsy: a study in ten patients. J Neurol 1992;239:284.
37. Feely M, Calvert R, Gibson J. Clobazam in catamenial epilepsy: a model for evaluating anticonvulsants. Lancet 1982;2:71.
38. Feely M, Gibson J. Intermittent clobazam for catamenial epilepsy: tolerance avoided. J Neurol Neurosurg Psychiatr 1984;47:1279.
39. Taylor DC. Sexual behavior and temporal lobe epilepsy. Arch Neurol 1969;21:510.
40. Morrell MJ, Sperling MR, Stecker M, et al. Sexual dysfunction in partial epilepsy: a deficit in physiologic sexual arousal. Neurology 1994;44:243.
41. Herzog AG, Seibel MM, Schomer DL, et al. Reproductive endocrine disorders in women with partial seizures of temporal lobe origin. Arch Neurol 1986;43:341.
42. Isojarvi JI, Laatikainen TJ, Pakarinen AJ, et al. Polycystic ovaries and hyperandrogenism in women taking valproate for epilepsy. N Engl J Med 1993;329:1383.
43. Isojarvi JI, Laatikainen TJ, Knip M, et al. Obesity and endocrine disorders in women taking valproate for epilepsy. Ann Neurol 1996;39:579.
44. Herzog AG. A relationship between particular reproductive endocrine disorders and the laterality of epileptiform discharges in women with epilepsy. Neurology 1993;43:1907.

45. Bilo L, Meo R, Nappi C, et al. Reproductive endocrine disorders in women with primary generalized epilepsy. Epilepsia 1988;29:612.
46. Cummings LN, Giudice L, Morrell MJ. Ovulatory function in epilepsy. Epilepsia 1995;36:355.
47. Herzog AG, Russell V, Vaitukaitis JL, et al. Neuroendocrine dysfunction in temporal lobe epilepsy. Arch Neurol 1982;39:133.
48. Drislane FW, Coleman AE, Schomer DL, et al. Altered pulsatile secretion of luteinizing hormone in women with epilepsy. Neurology 1994;44:306.
49. Isojarvi JI. Serum steroid hormones and pituitary function in female epileptic patients during carbamazepine therapy. Epilepsia 1990;31:438.
50. Isojarvi JI, Laatikainen TJ, Pakarinen AJ, et al. Menstrual disorders in women with epilepsy receiving carbamazepine. Epilepsia 1995;36:676.
51. Levesque LA, Herzog AG, Seibel MM. The effect of phenytoin and carbamazepine on serum dehydroepiandrosterone sulfate in men and women who have partial seizures with temporal lobe involvement. J Clin Endocrinol Metab 1986;63:243.
52. Cleland PG. Risk-benefit assessment of anticonvulsants in women of childbearing potential. Drug Safety 1991;6:70.
53. Wilder BJ. Safety considerations in the use of antiepileptic drugs: the role of phenytoin in the clinical management of epilepsy. Today's Therapeutic Trends 1991;9:29.
54. Espir M, Walker ME, Lawson JP. Epilepsy and oral contraception. BMJ 1969;639:294.
55. Dana-Haeri J, Richens A. Effect of norethisterone on seizures associated with menstruation. Epilepsia 1983;24:377.
56. Coulam CB, Annegers JF. Do anticonvulsants reduce the efficacy of oral contraceptives? Epilepsia 1979;20:519.
57. Sonnen AE. Sodium valproate and the contraceptive pill. Br J Clin Pract Symposium 1988;27(Suppl):31.
58. Back DJ, Grimmer SFM, Orme MLE, et al. Evaluation of Committee on Safety of Medicines Yellow Card reports on oral contraceptive-drug interactions with anticonvulsants and antibiotics. Br J Clin Pharmacol 1988;25:527.
59. Back DJ, Bates M, Bowden A, et al. The interaction of phenobarbital and other anticonvulsants with oral contraceptive therapy. Contraception 1980;22:495.
60. Crawford P, Chadwick DJ, Martin C, et al. The interaction of phenytoin and carbamazepine with combined oral contraceptive steroids. Br J Clin Pharmacol 1990;30:892.
61. Patsalos PN, Duncan JS. Antiepileptic drugs. A review of clinically significant drug interactions. Drug Safety 1993;9:156.
62. Holdich T, Whiteman P, Orme M, et al. Effect of lamotrigine on the pharmacology of the combined oral contraceptive pill. Epilepsia 1991;32(Suppl 1):96.
63. Eldon MA, Underwood BA, Randinitis EJ, et al. Lack of effect of gabapentin on the pharmacokinetics of a norethindrone acetate/ethinyl estradiol–containing oral contraceptive. Neurology 1993;43:A307.

64. Crawford P, Chadwick D, Cleland P, et al. The lack of effect of sodium valproate on the pharmacokinetics of oral contraceptive steroids. Contraception 1986;33:23.
65. Fraser IS. Contraceptive choice for women with "risk factors." Drug Safety 1993;8:271.
66. O'Brien MD, Gilmour-White S. Epilepsy and pregnancy. BMJ 1993;307:492.
67. Mattson RH, Cramer JA, Darney PD, et al. Use of oral contraceptives by women with epilepsy. JAMA 1986;256:238.
68. Orme M, Cranford P, Back D. Contraception, Epilepsy, and Pharmacokinetics. In MR Trimble (ed), Women and Epilepsy. New York: Wiley, 1991;145.
69. Yerby MS, Devinsky O. Epilepsy and Pregnancy. In O Devinsky, E Feldmann, B Hainline (eds), Neurological Complications of Pregnancy. New York: Raven, 1994;45.
70. Nelson KB, Ellenberg JH. Maternal seizure disorder, outcome of pregnancy, and neurologic abnormalities in the children. Neurology 1982;32:1247.
71. Jagoda A, Riggio S. Emergency department approach to managing seizures in pregnancy. Ann Emerg Med 1991;20:80.
72. Bag S, Behari M, Ahuja GK, et al. Pregnancy and epilepsy. J Neurol 1989;236:311.
73. Knight AH, Rhind EG. Epilepsy and pregnancy: a study of 153 pregnancies in 59 patients. Epilepsia 1975;16:99.
74. Yerby MS, Friel PN, McCormick K. Antiepileptic drug disposition during pregnancy. Neurology 1992;42(4 Suppl 5):12.
75. Hiilesmaa VK. Pregnancy and birth in women with epilepsy. Neurology 1992;42(4 Suppl 5):8.
76. Delgado-Escueta AV, Janz D. Consensus guidelines: preconception counseling, management, and care of the pregnant woman with epilepsy. Neurology 1992;42(4 Suppl 5):149.
77. Dansky LV, Andermann E, Andermann F. Marriage and fertility in epileptic patients. Epilepsia 1980;21:261.
78. Webber MP, Hauser WA, Ottman R, et al. Fertility in persons with epilepsy: 1935–1974. Epilepsia 1986;27:746.
79. Bjerkedal T, Bahana SL. The course and outcome of pregnancy in women with epilepsy. Acta Obstet Gynecol Scand 1973;52:245.
80. Yerby MS. Pregnancy, teratogenesis, and epilepsy. Neurol Clin 1994;12:749.
81. Lindhout D, Omtzigt JG. Teratogenic effects of antiepileptic drugs: implications for the management of epilepsy in women of childbearing age. Epilepsia 1994;35(Suppl 4):S19.
82. Ferendelli JA. Discussion: the renaissance of rational polytherapy: the new generation of antiepileptic medications. Neurology 1995;45(Suppl 2):S35.
83. Aminoff MJ. Neurologic Disorders. In RK Creasy, R Resnick (eds), Maternal-Fetal Medicine. Philadelphia: Saunders, 1994;1071.
84. Roberts JM. Magnesium for preeclampsia and eclampsia. N Engl J Med 1995;333:250.
85. Lucas MJ, Leveno KJ, Cunningham FG. A comparison of magnesium sulfate with phenytoin for the prevention of eclampsia. N Engl J Med 1995;333:201.

86. The Eclampsia Trial Collaborative Group. Which anticonvulsant for women with eclampsia? Evidence from the Collaborative Eclampsia Trial. Lancet 1995;345:1455.

87. Kaneko S, Suzuki K, Sato T, et al. The Problems of Antiepileptic Medication in the Neonatal Period: Is Breast-Feeding Advisable? In D Janz, L Bossi, M Dam (eds), Epilepsy, Pregnancy, and the Child. New York: Raven, 1982;343.

CHAPTER 2

Stroke

Merit E. Cudkowicz

Cerebrovascular disease is one of the leading causes of disability and death in women in the United States [1, 2]. Specific conditions put women at higher risk for stroke, including hormonal therapy, pregnancy, the presence of antiphospholipid antibodies (APAs), rheumatologic disorders, and migraine headaches. In addition, women may respond differently to stroke prevention treatment than do men [2]. Recognition of features of stroke that are specific to women may lead to better recognition, prevention, and management of stroke in women [3].

Ischemic Stroke

Epidemiology

Forty percent of the approximately 500,000 patients who suffer a stroke each year are women [1]. The overall mortality rate from stroke is higher in women than in men [4], probably due to the older age of women at the time of their initial stroke. Approximately one-third of strokes in women occur after age 75 [5]. Strokes are more common in men than in women in all age groups except for those under 35 [2, 6]. The predominance of stroke in younger women is thought to be due to oral contraceptive (OCP) use and pregnancy. The predominance of stroke in men in the older age group is attributed to the earlier age of onset of atherosclerosis. After menopause, there is an increase in the frequency and severity of cerebral atherosclerosis in women [2]. Intracranial atherosclerosis is more common in women [7].

Risk Factors

The risk factors for stroke, with the exception of hormonal therapy and pregnancy, are similar for men and women. Hypertension is the leading risk factor in both sexes [8]. Cardiac disease is the second most common risk factor and accounts for approximately 20% of strokes [9]. Smoking increases the risk of ischemic cerebral infarction 2.5 times in women [10]. OCP use also increases the risk of stroke in women who smoke [8, 11, 12]. Transient ischemic attacks (TIAs), diabetes, age, OCP use, pregnancy, the presence of APAs, cerebral vasculitis, migraine headache, sickle-cell disease, and elevated fibrinogen concentration are also important risk factors for stroke [13, 14].

Hormone Therapy in Women

Exogenous estrogen preparations may increase the risk of stroke in women. Most studies that evaluated the risk of stroke in women taking OCPs were completed before the development of lower-dose estrogen pills [11, 15, 16]. Several well-designed epidemiologic studies conclude that OCP use increases the risk of stroke [11, 16–18]. For example, a case control study of women less than 40 years old found the relative risk of an occlusive stroke to be 4.4 (95% confidence interval [CI], 0.68–24.4) in women using OCPs [15]. The risk of stroke increases for women taking OCPs who are over age 35, hypertensive, or smokers [11]. While high-dose estrogen OCPs (80–100 µg estrogen) are probably associated with increased stroke risk, it is not yet certain whether this is true of the low-dose preparations (30–35 µg estrogen). OCPs with a high estrogen content are associated with a higher incidence of stroke than those with lower estrogen preparation [19, 20].

The incidence of stroke in users of low-dose OCPs was evaluated in a population-based case control study [20]. Fatal and nonfatal strokes were studied in women ages 15–44 who were members of the California Kaiser Permanente Medical Care Program. After adjustment for known stroke risk factors, the odds ratio for ischemic stroke among current users of OCPs (low-dose preparations) was 1.18 (95% CI, 0.54–2.59) compared with former OCP users and women who had never used OCPs. They concluded that low-dose estrogen OCPs do not appear to increase the risk of stroke. OCPs now in widespread use in the United States contain 30–35 µg estrogen. It is unclear exactly how high-dose OCP use causes an increased incidence of cerebral infarction. The increased risk of ischemic stroke with OCP use may be secondary to changes in the coagulation system, platelet function, and lipid metabolism [2]. It is recommended that women who have had an ischemic stroke while taking OCPs discontinue their use.

Although the use of OCPs with high estrogen content is a well-established risk factor for stroke in women, the risk of stroke with estrogen replacement therapy (ERT) in postmenopausal women is less clear. Several epidemiologic studies have evaluated the effect of ERT on stroke risk in postmenopausal women [10, 21–25]. The findings are not consistent. Some studies have found an increased risk for stroke among estrogen users [22], whereas others document a decreased risk [21, 26]. Additional studies suggest that ERT has no effect on stroke risk [10, 23, 27, 28]. The risk of estrogen/progestin combinations on stroke in women is unknown [23]. A complete evaluation for other possible causes is strongly recommended in women receiving ERT who present with ischemic stroke.

It is unclear exactly how ERT may protect against ischemic stroke. Atherosclerosis increases in women after menopause [25]. Daily use of 0.625 mg or 1.25 mg oral conjugated equine estrogen is associated with an approximately 10–14% increase in high-density lipoprotein cholesterol levels and a 4–8% reduction in low-density lipoprotein (LDL) cholesterol levels [29]. Unopposed oral estrogen also lowers total cholesterol levels [25, 30]. The addition of cyclic progestin may improve lipid measurements [26]. Estrogen may also reduce plaque formation by inhibition of LDL oxidation, preventing the conversion of macrophages to foam cells [31].

Pregnancy

Pregnancy is associated with an approximately 13-fold increase in the incidence of ischemic cerebral infarction [32]. One study found that 35% of strokes in women of childbearing age are associated with pregnancy [33]. The incidence of stroke during pregnancy has been estimated at 3.5 per 100,000 pregnant women per year [34]. A small study compared stroke rates during pregnancy with those of nonpregnant women and demonstrated only a small increase in risk during pregnancy [34].

Approximately 60% of ischemic strokes during pregnancy are caused by arterial occlusions. Cerebral infarctions are most common in the third trimester and the puerperium, with few cases occurring in the first trimester [35]. Emboli from the heart cause the majority of arterial infarctions [36]. The risk of cardiogenic emboli may increase during pregnancy because of third-trimester changes in the coagulation and fibrinolytic system and increases in blood viscosity and stasis. Emboli from the lower extremity or pelvic veins can pass through an atrial septal defect or a patent foramen ovale and lead to cerebral infarction [2]. Several congenital and acquired cardiac abnormalities can also predispose an individual to thrombosis. These include atrial septal defects, mitral valve prolapse (MVP), peripartum cardiomyopathy, or endocarditis [2]. A congestive cardiomyopathy of unknown etiology can occur during the third trimester and early postpartum period. Mural cardiac thrombi may form and lead to embolic cerebral infarction. Anticoagulation with heparin is recommended if a thrombus is present or if an ischemic event has occurred [2, 35]. Other causes of stroke during pregnancy include hypertension, diabetes, cerebral venous thrombosis (CVT), premature atherosclerosis, arterial dissection, moyamoya disease, Takayasu's disease, sickle-cell disease, thrombotic thrombocytopenic purpura [36], and amniotic, fat, or air emboli [32, 37].

Approximately one-third of cerebral infarctions during pregnancy are due to CVT. CVT typically occurs in the late third trimester or early postpartum period [32, 36]. The range of reported incidence of CVT is from one in 1,666 to one in 10,000 pregnancies [38]. Patients typically present with headache, nausea and vomiting, focal or generalized seizures, and focal neurologic signs. Magnetic resonance imaging can confirm the diagnosis of CVT. The best treatment for CVT is not clear. Treatment with heparin carries the potential risk of hemorrhagic infarction. However, a small randomized clinical trial concluded that anticoagulation is an effective treatment and improves neurologic outcome [39]. Anticoagulation is usually continued for 2–3 months [36]. Thrombolysis has been tried in at least one subject with postpartum CVT [40]. Thrombolytic therapy has not been adequately studied in pregnant patients; none of the currently available agents are recommended during pregnancy. The etiology of CVT is unclear; however, predisposing factors include dehydration and infections.

The evaluation of a pregnant patient who experiences a stroke is similar to that for a nonpregnant patient. However, pregnant patients should also be evaluated for choriocarcinoma, postpartum cardiomyopathy, and paradoxic emboli. In the treatment of stroke in pregnant women, medications should be carefully selected. Warfarin sodium (Coumadin) therapy crosses the placenta and is teratogenic when used during the first trimester of pregnancy. Heparin, which does not cross the placenta, is therefore recommended [41]. The following causes of stroke should be treated with heparin: cardiac emboli, presence of APAs, and clinically progressive CVT. Low-dose aspirin (60–80 mg per day) can be used during pregnancy for preventing ischemic stroke in women with an appropriate risk factor [36, 42].

Antiphospholipid Antibodies

APAs and the associated risk of cerebral ischemia are more common in women than men. APAs are circulating serum polyclonal immunoglobulins that bind negatively charged phospholipids [2]. Several studies have reported the association between APAs and stroke [43]. APAs, including anticardiolipin antibodies and the lupus anticoagulant, are independent risk factors for ischemic stroke. Anticardiolipin antibodies have been reported in 6.8–29.0% of patients with ischemic stroke [43]. The IgG anticardiolipin antibody is the predominant antibody associated with an increased stroke risk [44]. Risk factors for the presence of this antibody include being young or female, experiencing recurrent first-trimester spontaneous abortion, and having had prior TIAs or strokes [44]. Patients with APAs suffer stroke or TIAs at a younger age than the general stroke population [45, 46]. Brey and colleagues found that 45.6% of stroke or TIA patients under age 50 had APAs. Mean age at onset of stroke was 42.6 years (standard deviation 14.8); the female-to-male ratio was 4 to 1 [46, 47]. There is also an increased risk of multiple strokes with recurrence rates ranging from 6.75% to 36% [44].

APAs are frequently detected in young women with systemic lupus erythematosus (SLE) [48]. Approximately 50% of patients treated for SLE have APAs. In patients with SLE, the incidence of arterial and venous thromboses ranges from 20% to 36% [49, 50]. APAs are also present in patients with malignancy, leukemia, immune thrombocytopenia purpura, infection, Lyme disease, syphilis, and Behçet's disease, as well as those treated with chlorpromazine and procainamide. APAs increase the risk of ischemic stroke and fetal complications during pregnancy [51]. There is a primary APA syndrome that is defined by the presence of APA or lupus anticoagulant, and any or all of the following: recurrent thromboses, recurrent fetal losses, and thrombocytopenia. This syndrome is also more common in young women and is associated primarily with high titers of IgG anticardiolipin antibody.

Due to the high incidence of recurrent stroke, the use of low-dose warfarin sodium in young nonpregnant women with ischemic stroke related to APAs has been recommended. Subcutaneous heparin should be considered in pregnant women with APAs who develop symptoms of cerebral ischemia. Preventive therapy for patients who have not had clinical symptoms is controversial.

Cerebral Vasculitis

Cerebral vasculitis occurs in several of the systemic vasculitides including polyarteritis nodosa, Wegener's granulomatosis, Behçet's disease, Takayasu's disease, SLE, mixed connective tissue disease, rheumatoid arthritis (RA), and Sjögren's syndrome [52]. Cerebral infarction and hemorrhage are rare outcomes. A female predominance is present in Takayasu's disease, SLE, RA, and Sjögren's syndrome [52]. Symptoms of both SLE and Takayasu's disease may worsen during pregnancy and the postpartum period [6, 32]. Other causes of cerebral vasculitis affect men and women similarly, including those associated with infectious agents, neoplasms, cocaine, and amphetamines [3, 53].

A small-vessel angiopathy is present in patients with SLE. Clinical presentation often includes multiple cerebral infarctions, encephalopathy, and seizures. Exacerbation of symptoms occurs frequently during pregnancy and may cause an increased risk of fetal death. Exacerbation of SLE during pregnancy is treated with steroids for the remainder of the pregnancy and for 2 months postpartum. A large-vessel angiopathy affecting the aortic arch and its branches is found with Takayasu's arteritis. Clinical presentation often includes symptoms of retinopathy and multiple cerebral infarctions. Exacerbation is commonly seen during pregnancy [6].

Migraine Headache

Approximately 25% of women suffer from migraine headaches [3]. It has not been definitively determined whether migraine headache is an independent risk factor for stroke. Migraine may increase the risk of stroke in association with other stroke risk factors such as smoking and OCP use. The Collaborative Group for the Study of Stroke in Young Women suggests that the relative risk for thrombotic stroke in women with migraine was twice that in controls [11]. The posterior circulation is the most commonly affected vascular distribution [54]. The diagnosis of migraine-related stroke requires exclusion of all other known causes of stroke, a history of migraines, and occurrence during a typical migraine attack. Cerebral angiograms are typically normal. If performed during an attack, cerebral angiograms are associated with an increased risk of complications [54].

Treatment for women who have had a stroke related to migraine is daily aspirin; migraine prophylaxis with calcium antagonists or tricyclic antidepressants are recommended [3]. Ergotamines and sumatriptan should be avoided [2]. In addition, modification of high-risk factors including discontinuation of smoking and OCP use is recommended. The pathogenesis of stroke in migraine is unknown. Vasospasm, increased platelet aggregation, and impaired platelet function have been implicated [2].

Mitral Valve Prolapse

An association between MVP and cerebral ischemic events has been found in several studies [3, 55]. MVP is a common cardiac abnormality. The estimated prevalence is between 5% and 15%, with a female preponderance [3]. It is associated with 1.25% of strokes in older adults and 0.02% of strokes in adults less than 40 years old. TIAs associated with MVP are more common than cerebral infarction. The diagnosis of MVP-associated cerebral ischemia and infarction is a diagnosis of exclusion after all other possible causes have been eliminated. Stroke prophylactic treatment is not recommended in asymptomatic patients. The etiology of MVP-associated stroke is probably cardiogenic emboli.

Stroke Prevention

Aspirin and ticlopidine are antiplatelet agents that reduce the risk of recurrent stroke. Results from several stroke prevention trials suggest that aspirin is more effective for men than for women [8, 56–59]. However, other studies have found no gender differences in the effects of aspirin on stroke prevention [60–62]. For example, subgroup analysis of a European stroke prevention study found that antiplatelet therapy is as effective in women as in men in the prevention of stroke or death. The combination of dipyridamole, 75 mg tid, and acetylsalicylic acid, 330 mg tid, was compared to placebo use for the secondary prevention of stroke or death after one or more recent attacks of TIA or stroke of atherothrombotic origin.

Forty-five percent of 2,500 subjects were women. End-point reduction compared with the placebo group in the treatment group was about 50% in women and 40% in men [62].

The gender difference in response to aspirin may reflect the small number of women tested in each of these clinical studies; however, it may also represent a true gender difference in the antiplatelet effects of aspirin. Results from Spranger and colleagues suggest that aspirin may have a different effect on platelets based on gender. They studied whole-blood platelet aggregation in healthy men and women and in men with carcinoma of the prostate who had orchiectomy. The in vitro inhibitory effect of aspirin on spontaneous platelet aggregation was significantly greater in men than in postmenopausal women or orchiectomized men [63].

Stroke prevention trials using ticlopidine have found equal benefit in women and men [57, 64, 65]. The Ticlopidine Aspirin Stroke Study compared the effects of 500 mg per day of ticlopidine to 1,300 mg per day of aspirin in 3,069 patients with a recent TIA or minor stroke [64]. The risk reduction in recurrent stroke was similar for women and men. In another study, ticlopidine, 250 mg bid, was compared with aspirin, 650 mg bid, in 4,069 patients with a recent TIA or mild stroke. There was no significant difference in response to ticlopidine based on gender, though there was a trend toward an increased response in women. The risk reduction for fatal or nonfatal stroke was 27% for women compared with 19% for men [64]. Adverse effects of ticlopidine include diarrhea, rash, and reversible severe neutropenia. Because of these adverse effects, ticlopidine is only recommended for patients who are unable to take aspirin.

Carotid Endarterectomy for Patients with Carotid Disease

It is unknown whether a gender difference in response to carotid endarterectomy for asymptomatic carotid artery stenosis exists. The Asymptomatic Carotid Artery Study randomly assigned 1,662 asymptomatic patients, including 535 women, to either the best medical care plus endarterectomy or to the best medical care only [66]. There was an overall 53% relative risk reduction of stroke with carotid endarterectomy [67]. Post-hoc subgroup analysis found a statistically insignificant difference in 5-year relative-risk reduction between men and women [66].

Intracerebral Hemorrhage

Epidemiology

Intracerebral hemorrhage (ICH) occurs with equal frequency in men and women. However, subarachnoid hemorrhage (SAH) from a ruptured aneurysm is more common in women by a ratio of 1.5 to 1 [68]. Women are also twice as likely to have a recurrent SAH from an aneurysm within 2 weeks of the initial event and have four times the mortality rate from SAH of men [69]. The reasons for the differences in incidence, recurrence rate, and mortality rate are unknown. A possible role for hormones has been suggested by studies that found exogenous hormonal therapy and pregnancy to be associated with increased risk of SAH [15].

Hormone Therapy

The exact risk of SAH with various hormonal therapies is unknown. The risk of SAH may be increased in OCP users; however, there are also studies that find no increased risk [15]. A study found an association between OCP use and smoking with the risk of hemorrhagic strokes. The odds ratio for women with both risk factors was 3.64 (95% CI, 0.95–13.87) [20]. The risk of SAH in patients receiving ERT may be reduced by 40–50%; however, other studies have not found similar effects [26].

Pregnancy

Rupture of an aneurysm or arteriovenous malformation (AVM) is the most common cause of ICH during pregnancy [70]. Clinical presentation includes abrupt onset of a severe headache with altered levels of consciousness, seizures, and focal neurologic signs. The maternal mortality rate is 35% after an aneurysmal hemorrhage and 28% after an AVM hemorrhage [71]. Recurrent bleeding during the remainder of pregnancy from an untreated aneurysm or AVM is estimated to occur in 33–50% of patients, with a maternal mortality rate of 50–68% [71]. Other causes of ICH during pregnancy include CVT, severe hypertension, drug abuse, thrombocytopenia, anticoagulation treatment, and metastatic choriocarcinoma [72].

Intracranial aneurysm rupture occurs five times more often in pregnant than in nonpregnant women [72, 73]. The peak risk of aneurysm rupture is from 30–40 weeks gestation to 2–6 weeks postpartum. The outcome is worse for the mother and infant if the aneurysm is untreated, secondary to higher rates of rebleeding and fatality [74]. Women with AVMs have a 10% risk of ICH; this risk increases to 87% during pregnancy [72, 74]. The maternal mortality rate from an AVM hemorrhage during pregnancy is 28% compared to 10% in a nonpregnant woman [71]. The risk of recurrent hemorrhage is 27% during the same pregnancy with a 26% risk of fetal death [72, 74].

The management of aneurysmal SAH and AVMs during pregnancy is very difficult. Early referral to an experienced clinical center and neurosurgeon is crucial. Intensive care facilities are equipped to treat cerebral vasospasm and edema. Nimodipine is a cerebroselective calcium antagonist that is used to prevent complications of cerebral vasospasm after aneurysm rupture [75]. Its safety in pregnancy is unknown. Early neurosurgical treatment after aneurysmal hemorrhage [71, 76] is currently recommended. The advantage of early operative intervention after aneurysmal hemorrhage during pregnancy was examined by Dias and Sekhar in 106 patients who suffered aneurysmal hemorrhage before delivery. Fifty-five received operative treatment during pregnancy, and 51 were not treated surgically. Both maternal and fetal mortality were significantly lower for patients whose aneurysms were treated operatively. Maternal mortality was 11% in the group treated operatively and 63% in the group not treated, while fetal mortality was 5% in the group treated operatively and 27% in the group not treated [71]. The optimal management of pregnant patients with a known cerebral aneurysm that has not ruptured is not clearly established.

The correct surgical management of a ruptured AVM during pregnancy is not clear. In the same study by Dias and Sekhar there was no statistical difference in maternal or fetal mortality in the group treated operatively compared with the group treated medically [71]. It is recommended that decisions regarding surgical management of an AVM during pregnancy should be the same in both pregnant and nonpregnant patients. For patients with unresected lesions, the risk of intracranial bleeding during vaginal delivery is not significantly different from that associated with cesarean section [71].

The reasons that aneurysms and AVMs bleed with increasing frequency in the latter trimesters are not known. It is possible that the hemodynamic changes of pregnancy may predispose an individual to ICH [71].

Conclusion

Several characteristics unique to women influence the prevention, etiology, treatment, and outcome of stroke in women. A variety of conditions predispose women to an increased risk of stroke, including hormonal therapy, pregnancy, the presence of APAs, systemic vasculitides, and migraine headaches. Optimal management of stroke in women is still unclear. Although anticoagulation is recommended for ischemic stroke, the effectiveness of antiplatelet therapy is not certain.

References

1. Love B. Stroke in women. Hawaii Med J 1994;53:258.
2. Knepper L, Giuliani M. Cerebrovascular disease in women. Cardiology 1995;86:339.
3. Wong M, Guiliani M, Haley E. Cerebrovascular disease and stroke in women. Cardiology 1990;77(Suppl 2):80.
4. Bonita R. Epidemiology of stroke. Lancet 1992;339:344.
5. Sacco R, Hauser W, Mohr J. Hospitalized stroke in blacks and hispanics in northern Manhattan. Stroke 1991;22:1491.

6. Bogousslavsky J, Pierre P. Ischemic stroke in patients under age 45. Neurol Clin 1992;10:113.
7. Caplan L, Gorelick P, Hier D. Race, sex and occlusive cerebrovascular disease: a review. Stroke 1986;17:648.
8. Hershey L. Stroke prevention in women: role of aspirin versus ticlopidine. Am J Med 1991;91:288.
9. Wolf P, Abbott R, Kannel W. Atrial fibrillation: a major contributor to stroke in the elderly. Arch Intern Med 1987;147:1561.
10. Thompson S, Greenbert G, Meade T. Risk factors for stroke and myocardial infarction in women in the United Kingdom as assessed in general practice: a case-control study. Br Heart J 1989;61:403.
11. Collaborative Group for the Study of Stroke in Young Women. Oral contraceptives and stroke in young women. JAMA 1975;231:718.
12. Layde P, Beral V, Kay C. Royal College of General Practitioners Oral Contraceptive Study. Lancet 1981;1:541.
13. Wolf P, Belanger A, D'Agostino R. Management of risk factors. Neurol Clin 1992;10:177.
14. The Antiphospholipid in Stroke Study (APASS) Group. Anticardiolipin antibodies are an independent risk factor for first ischemic stroke. Neurology 1993;43:2069.
15. Thorogood M, Mann J, Murphy M, et al. Fatal stroke and use of oral contraceptives: findings from a case-control study. Am J Epidemiol 1992;136:35.
16. Collaborative Group for the Study of Stroke in Young Women. Oral contraception and increased risk of cerebral ischemia or thrombosis. N Engl J Med 1973;288:871.
17. Vessey M, Doll R. Investigation of relation between use of oral contraceptives and thromboembolic disease: a further report. BMJ 1969;2:651.
18. Sartwell P, Masi A, Arthes F, et al. Thromboembolisms and oral contraceptives: an epidemiologic case-control study. Am J Epidemiol 1969;90:365.
19. Battenger L. Oral contraceptives and thromboembolic disease: effects of lowering estrogen content. Lancet 1980;1:1097.
20. Petitti D, Sidney S, Bernstein A, et al. Stroke in users of low-dose oral contraceptives. N Engl J Med 1996;335:8.
21. Ross R, Pike M, Henderson B, et al. Stroke prevention and estrogen replacement therapy. Lancet 1989;1:505.
22. Wilson P, Garrison R, Castelli W. Postmenopausal estrogen use, cigarette smoking and cardiovascular morbidity in women over 50. N Engl J Med 1985;313:1038.
23. Grady D, Rubin S, Petitti D, et al. Review: hormone therapy to prevent disease and prolong life in postmenopausal women. Ann Intern Med 1992;117:1016.
24. Stampfer M, Coldtiz G, Willett W, et al. Postmenopausal estrogen therapy and cardiovascular disease. N Engl J Med 1991;325:756.
25. Belchetz P. Hormonal treatment of post-menopausal women. N Engl J Med 1994;330:1062.

26. Paganini-Hill A. Estrogen replacement therapy and stroke. Prog Cardiovasc Dis 1995;38:223.
27. Rosenberg S, Fausone V, Clark R. The role of estrogens as a risk factor for stroke in postmenopausal women. West J Med 1980;133:292.
28. Pfeffer R, Van der Noort S. Estrogen use and stroke risk in postmenopausal women. Am J Epidemiol 1976;103:445.
29. Bush T, Miller V. Effects of Pharmacologic Agents Used During Menopause: Impact on Lipid and Lipoproteins. In D Mishell (ed), Menopause: Physiology and Pharmacology. Chicago: Year Book, 1987;187.
30. Walsh B, Schiff I, Rosner B, et al. Effects of postmenopausal estrogen replacement on the concentrations and metabolisms of plasma lipoproteins. N Engl J Med 1991;325:1196.
31. Sack M, Rader D, Cannon RI. Estrogen and inhibition of oxidation of low-density lipoprotein in postmenopausal women. Atherosclerosis 1994;89:175.
32. Wiebers D. Ischemic cerebrovascular complications of pregnancy. Arch Neurol 1985;42:1106.
33. Jennett W, Cross J. Influence of pregnancy and oral contraception on the incidence of stroke in women of childbearing age. Lancet 1967;1:1019.
34. Wiebers D, Whisnant J. The incidence of stroke among pregnant women in Rochester, Minn, 1955–1979. JAMA 1985;254:3055.
35. Simolke G, Cox S, Cunningham F. Cerebrovascular accidents complicating pregnancy and the puerperium. Obstet Gynecol 1991;78:37.
36. Donaldson J, Lee N. Arterial and venous stroke associated with pregnancy. Neurology Clin 1994;3:583.
37. Cunningham F, Leveno K. Management of Pregnancy-Induced Hypertension. In P Rubin (ed), Handbook of Hypertension. Oxford: Elsevier, 1988;209.
38. Carroll J, Leak D, Lee H. Cerebral thrombophlebitis in pregnancy and the puerperium. Q J Med 1966;35:347.
39. Villringer A, Garner C, Meister W, et al. High-dose heparin treatment in cerebral sinus-venous thrombosis. Stroke 1988;19:135.
40. DiRocco C, Iannelli A, Leone G. Heparin-urokinase treatment in aseptic dural sinus thrombosis. Arch Neurol 1981;38:431.
41. Ginsberg J, Hirsh J. Use of antithrombotic agents during pregnancy. Chest 1992;102:385.
42. Sibai B, Mirro R, Chesney C, et al. Low-dose aspirin in pregnancy. Obstet Gynecol 1989;74:551.
43. Montalban J, Codina A, Ordi J, et al. Antiphospholipid antibodies in cerebral ischemia. Stroke 1991;22:750.
44. Levine S, Welch K. Cerebrovascular ischemia associated with lupus anticoagulant. Stroke 1987;18:257.
45. Babikian V, Gorelick P, Kelley R. The lupus anticoagulant and stroke: clinical features. Neurology 1987;37:85.
46. Orefice G, Ames P, Coppola M, et al. Antiphospholipid antibodies and cerebrovascular disease. Acta Neurol 1993;15:303.

47. Brey R, Hart R, Sherman D, et al. Antiphospholipid antibodies and cerebral ischemia in young people. Neurology 1990;40:1190.
48. Lockshin M. Antiphospholipid antibody syndrome. JAMA 1992;268:1451.
49. Loizou S, Cofiner C, Weetman A, et al. Immunoglobulin class and IgG subclass distributions of anticardiolipin antibodies in patients with systemic lupus erythematosus and associated disorders. Clin Exp Immunol 1992;92:434.
50. Brenner B, Tavor S, Lerner M, et al. Association of lupus anticoagulant and anticardiolipin antibodies with thrombosis in patients with systemic lupus erythematosus, primary antiphospholipid syndrome and other disorders. Isr J Med Sci 1992;28:9.
51. Lockwood C, Romero R, Feinberg R, et al. The prevalence and biologic significance of lupus anticoagulant and anticardiolipin antibodies in a general obstetric population. Am J Obstet Gynceol 1989;161:369.
52. Sigal L. The neurologic presentation of vasculitic and rheumatologic syndromes: a review. Medicine 1987;66:157.
53. Merkel P, Koroshetz W, Irizarry M, et al. Cocaine-associated cerebral vasculitis. Semin Arthritis Rheumatol 1995;25:172.
54. Welch K, Levine S. Migraine-related stroke in the context of the International Headache Society Classification of Head Pain. Arch Neurol 1990;47:458.
55. Barnett H. Transient cerebral ischemia: pathogenesis, prognosis and management. Ann R Coll Physicians Surg Can 1974;7:153.
56. Canadian Cooperative Study Group. A randomized trial of aspirin and sulfinpyrazone in threatened stroke. N Engl J Med 1978;299:53.
57. Vike J. Stroke and its effect in women. JAMA 1994;49:198.
58. ISIS-2 (Second International Study of Infarct Survival) Collaborative Group. Randomised trial of intravenous streptokinase, oral aspirin, both or neither among 17,187 cases of suspected acute myocardial infarction, ISIS-2. Lancet 1988;2:349.
59. UK-TIA Group. United Kingdom Transient Ischemic Attack (UK-TIA) Aspirin Trial: interim results. BMJ 1988;296:316.
60. Bousser M, Eschwege E, Haguenau M, et al. AICLA controlled trial of aspirin and dipyridamole in the secondary prevention of atherothrombotic cerebral ischemia. Stroke 1983;14:5.
61. American-Canadian Cooperative Study Group. Persantine aspirin trial in cerebral ischemia. Part II. Endpoint results. Stroke 1985;16:406.
62. Sivenius J, Riekkinen P, Kilpelainene H, et al. Antiplatelet therapy is effective in the prevention of stroke or death in women: subgroup analysis of the European Stroke Prevention Study (ESPS). Acta Neurol Scand 1991;84:286.
63. Spranger M, Aspey B, Harrison M. Sex difference in antithrombotic effect of aspirin. Stroke 1989;20:34.
64. Hass W, Easton J, Adams H, et al. A randomized trial comparing ticlopidine hydrochloride with aspirin for the prevention of stroke in high-risk patients. N Engl J Med 1989;321:501.
65. Gent M, Blakely J, Easton D, et al. The Canadian American Ticlopidine Study (CATS) in thromboembolic stroke. Lancet 1989;1:1215.

66. Barnett H, Meldrun H, Eliasziw M. Perspectives: the dilemma of surgical treatment for patients with asymptomatic carotid disease. Ann Intern Med 1995;123:723.
67. Executive Committee for the Asymptomative Carotid Atherosclerosis Study. Endarterectomy for asymptomatic carotid artery stenosis. JAMA 1995;273:1421.
68. Kurtzke J. Epidemiology of Cerebrovascular Disease. In F McDowell, L Caplan (eds), Cerebrovascular Survey Report 1985. National Institute of Neurological and Communicative Disorders and Stroke, National Institutes of Health, Public Health Service, 1985;1.
69. Torner J, Kassell N, Wallace R, et al. Preoperative prognostic factors for rebleeding and survival in aneurysm patients receiving antifibrinolytic therapy: report of the Cooperative Aneurysm Study. Neurosurgery 1981;9:506.
70. Barno A, Freedman D. Maternal deaths due to spontaneous subarachnoid hemorrhage. Am J Obstet Gynecol 1976;82:192.
71. Dias M, Sekhar L. Intracranial hemorrhage from aneurysms and arteriovenous malformations during pregnancy and the puerperium. Neurosurgery 1990;27:855.
72. Wiebers D. Subarachnoid hemorrhage in pregnancy. Semin Neurol 1988;8:226.
73. Fox M, Harms R, Davis D. Selected neurologic complications of pregnancy. Mayo Clin Proc 1990;65:1595.
74. Robinson J, Hall C, Sedzimir C. Arteriovenous malformations, aneurysms and pregnancy. J Neurosurg 1974;41:63.
75. Wong M, Haley E. Calcium antagonists: stroke therapy coming of age. Curr Concepts Cerebrovasc Dis Stroke 1989;24:31.
76. Schwartz J. Pregnancy complicated by subarachnoid hemorrhage. Am J Obstet Gynecol 1951;62:539.

CHAPTER 3

Headache Syndromes

F. Michael Cutrer

Headaches are among the most common complaints encountered by physicians. A large-scale epidemiologic study of adults indicated that 78% of women and 68% of men in the United States suffer from headaches [1]. Many common headache syndromes, such as migraine and tension-type headache (TTH), disproportionately affect women. Almost 18% of women in the United States meet the clinical criteria for the diagnosis of migraine headaches, while just under 6% of men do [2]. A significant proportion of migraineurs experience moderate to severe disability during the course of illness. Migraine and other headache syndromes exact a high cost in suffering and lost productivity on the affected individual, their families, and coworkers.

Headaches are categorized either as secondary headaches, which are symptomatic of an identifiable underlying abnormality, or as primary headaches, which occur in the absence of such an abnormality. Although this discussion focuses on the diagnosis and management of primary disorders, which constitute the overwhelming majority of headaches, pseudotumor cerebri, a secondary headache disorder commonly occurring in women, is also reviewed.

Etiology of Headaches

Surgery performed on the brains of awake epilepsy patients over 50 years ago provides very important information about the origins of headache. These procedures demonstrated that electrical or mechanical stimulation of the meninges or the blood vessels supplying them resulted in severe, throbbing head pain on the side of stimulation while similar stimulation of the brain itself caused no such pain [3]. These observations and subsequent investigations indicate that the meningeal vessels and meninges are very important structures in the genesis of headache. Meningeal and cerebral vessels are richly supplied with small-caliber sensory neurons called *C fibers*. On depolarization, C fibers from the meninges transmit the pain information within the trigeminal nerve, through the trigeminal ganglion (which contains the cell bodies of these neurons), and into the trigeminal nucleus caudalis (TNC) in the lower medulla [4]. Within the TNC the pain information is modulated by inhibitory interneurons and descending cortical inhibitory systems. From the caudal brain stem, fibers carrying the nociceptive signals project to more rostral trigeminal subnuclei and the thalamus. Projections from the thalamus ascend to the cerebral cortex, where pain information is localized and reaches consciousness.

In addition to the central transmission of pain, depolarization of the meningeal C fibers results in the release of vasoactive neuropeptide substances from activated C fiber terminals. Increasing evidence indicates that the released neuropeptides, including substance P, neurokinin A, and calcitonin–gene-related peptide, mediate a sterile inflammatory process within the meninges that in turn lowers the thresholds within the activated neurons for subsequent reactivation. This inflammation may be the mechanism by which headaches can continue on for hours or days and may also explain the effectiveness of anti-inflammatory drugs in many headache syndromes [5].

Primary Headache Disorders

Primary headache disorders, which occur without an identifiable abnormality as their cause, are very common in the general population and exceedingly common in women. The International Headache Society (IHS) has established diagnostic criteria for primary headache disorders based on clinical features of individual episodes. These criteria facilitate differentiation of the headache syndromes and thereby allow for more effective treatment. Two of the three major primary headache disorders (TTH and migraine) and one of the minor syndromes (chronic paroxysmal hemicrania) occur more commonly in women than in men. The reason for this female predominance is not well understood. Proposed explanations include gender-based differences in reporting of symptoms, use of health care, social roles, and perception of bodily sensations [6]. It is even more likely that hormonal fluctuations associated with menstruation act as potent triggers that generate headache in women. However, the mechanisms by which this occurs are still under investigation.

Tension-Type Headache

TTH is the most common primary headache disorder. Estimates of its prevalence range from 40% to 78% [7, 8]. TTH is less likely to result in visits to physicians, probably due to the relatively moderate pain intensity and general responsiveness to over-the-counter remedies. Both population- and clinic-based epidemiologic studies indicate that women are more likely to suffer from TTH than men [7–11]. Although the female predominance has been attributed to various gender-related psychological differences, a population-based study indicated that female predominance in TTH could not be explained by gender differences in psychometric testing [12].

The origin of TTH and the role of muscle contraction in its pathophysiology are still not understood. The presence of pericranial muscle spasm or tenderness is not necessary for the diagnosis. TTH occurs in both episodic and chronic forms. To fulfill the IHS diagnostic criteria for TTH, patients must have had at least 10 headaches that last from 30 minutes to 7 days and have at least two of the following characteristics: a pressing or tightening (nonthrobbing) quality, mild or moderate intensity, bilateral location, and no aggravation experienced with routine physical activity. In addition, they cannot be associated with nausea, vomiting, or any other physical abnormality. They may be associated with either photophobia or phonophobia, but not both [13].

Acute Treatment of Tension-Type Headache

The majority of patients with TTH need only acute treatment and use nonprescription medications quite effectively. However, a subgroup experiences frequent or refractory TTHs and requires daily prophylactic treatment for a period of time. Acute treatments for TTH include the following medications:

1.   Nonsteroidal anti-inflammatory drugs (NSAIDs) are the mainstay of the acute treatment of TTH. NSAIDs can exert analgesic, anti-inflammatory, and antipyretic effects through the inhibition of cyclooxygenase. Cyclooxygenase inhibition blocks the formation of proinflammatory prostaglandins as well as the aggregation of platelets. NSAIDs commonly used in TTH include aspirin, ibuprofen, ketoprofen, naproxen, naproxen sodium, ketorolac tromethamine, and indomethacin. Side effects of NSAIDs include dyspepsia, diarrhea, gastritis, increased bleeding time, and, with long-term, high-dose use, renal abnormalities. With toxic levels, tinnitus can occur. Contraindications include peptic ulcer disease, hypersensitivity to other NSAIDs, chronic anticoagulation therapy, and renal or liver disease.

2.   Acetaminophen in both 650- and 1,000-mg doses is often effective in the treatment of moderate TTH. Severe headaches are less likely to respond to acetaminophen. Gastric side effects are much less prominent than with NSAIDs. Toxic levels of acetaminophen can result in hepatic damage, and chronic, long-term use can lead to renal damage.

3.   Muscle relaxants are sometimes used to treat TTH. In theory, these agents relax pericranial muscles and thereby alleviate pain. In prac-

tice, these treatments are usually disappointing. Muscle relaxants some-times used in TTH include baclofen, dantrolene sodium, and cyclobenza-prine hydrochloride. There are no controlled clinical trials indicating efficacy of these agents in the treatment of acute TTH, and their use is largely empiric.

Prophylactic Treatment of Tension-Type Headache

Tricyclic antidepressants are the first-line agents in the prophylactic treat-ment of TTH. Although their exact mechanism is not known, the tricyclic antidepressants may suppress nociceptive neurotransmission through an inhibition of serotonin (5-HT) and norepinephrine reuptake. Of the tri-cyclics, the tertiary amine amitriptyline is the drug of choice. Amitripty-line at doses of 10–75 mg has been shown to be effective in double-blind, placebo-controlled studies [14]. Its use can be limited by sedation and anti-cholinergic side effects, such as dry mouth, tachycardia, constipation, or urinary retention. It should be started at a low dosage (10 mg per day) and slowly increased over several weeks (10-mg increments at intervals of 1–2 weeks). Beneficial effects may not be seen for 4–6 weeks. Other tricyclic antidepressants such as nortriptyline, desipramine, or imipramine may be useful. At present, however, there is very little evidence of their efficacy in clinical trials.

Maprotiline, a tetracyclic antidepressant, decreased headache severity by 25% and increased headache-free days by 40% in a small, double-blind, placebo-controlled study [15]. Dosages of 25–150 mg per day are used to treat depression. Low doses can be tried in headache patients.

Doxepin improved TTH in a small double-blind study [16]. Dosages from 10 to 150 mg per day are used. Side effects are similar to amitriptyline.

Fluoxetine, a selective serotonin-reuptake inhibitor, was reported in a small, open study to be effective in the treatment of TTH [17].

NSAIDs are clearly first-line agents in the acute treatment of TTH; however, at present, there are no studies of their effectiveness in prophylaxis.

Migraine Headache

Migraine headache is one of the most common maladies to afflict women. Migraine falls into two categories: migraine without aura (previously called *common migraine*), and migraine with aura (previously called *clas-sic migraine*). Prodromal symptoms, which include hyperactivity, eupho-ria, lethargy, depression, and thirst or food cravings, begin 24–48 hours before a headache in many patients. These symptoms should not be con-fused with the migraine aura, which is characterized by focal neurologic symptoms that occur within 1 hour of the onset of the headache. The headache phase is similar in both migraine with and without aura.

To fulfill the IHS's diagnostic criteria for migraine without aura, a patient must have had at least five attacks lasting 4–72 hours that have at least two of the following characteristics: unilateral location, pulsating quality, moderate or severe intensity, and aggravation with routine physical activity. In addition, these attacks are often associated with nausea, vomiting, photophobia, and phonophobia. They are not correlated with any other physical abnormality [13].

For the diagnosis of migraine with aura, in addition to fulfilling the criteria of migraine without aura, patients must have had at least two attacks with three of the four following characteristics:

1. Attacks are associated with reversible aura symptoms indicating focal cerebral cortical dysfunction, brain stem dysfunction, or both.
2. At least one of the aura symptoms develops gradually over 4 minutes or two or more symptoms occur in succession.
3. No aura symptom lasts for more than 1 hour. If more than one aura symptom is present, the accepted duration is increased accordingly.
4. Headache follows resolution of aura symptoms within 1 hour or less. (Headache can sometimes begin simultaneously with the aura.)

In addition, neither the headache nor the aura symptoms can be correlated to another physical abnormality.

Migraine aura symptoms can include homonymous visual disturbance, classically presenting as a scintillating scotoma; unilateral paresthesias and numbness; unilateral weakness; aphasia or other language disturbance; and nonvertiginous dizziness.

In patients with basilar migraine, the aura symptoms localize to the brain stem. These symptoms include decreased level of consciousness, ataxia, double vision, tinnitus, decreased hearing, vertigo, dysarthria, bilateral paresthesias or tingling, bilateral weakness, and visual symptoms in the temporal and nasal fields of both eyes. Some of these symptoms, such as bilateral tingling in the hands or dizziness, are subject to misinterpretation and can occur with anxiety or hyperventilation. In many patients, basilar attacks are intermingled with typical attacks. Basilar migraine was first described and most commonly occurs in young women [18, 19].

In complicated migraine, the aura symptoms persist after the headache for no longer than 1 week, and neuroimaging studies are normal.

In familial hemiplegic migraine, the aura includes hemiparesis. For the diagnosis, at least one first-degree relative must have similar attacks. This form of migraine has been localized to chromosome 19 in several families [20].

Menstrual Migraine

The cyclic hormonal fluctuations that accompany the menstrual cycle are a known trigger for migraine attacks in many women. Studies in school children by Bille found that the prevalence of migraine increases from the ages of 6 to 15 but that before age 11 (the average age of menarche), no female predominance is present [21]. Estimates of menstruation-associated migraine range from 10% to 70% of all migraine in women [22, 23]. In the 1960s, Lance and Anthony reported that in a large study of headache patients, 60% of female migraineurs linked at least some of their attacks to their menstrual cycle [24]. However, if a more rigid definition of menstrual migraine is applied, in which attacks are without aura and occur during the week before or during menstruation, then the occurrence rate drops to a much lower range of 8–14% [25, 26]. Those women who meet the rigid definition of menstrual migraine appear to be more likely to have had the onset of their migraine with menarche and to experience improvement in their migraine with pregnancy [26]. Menstrual migraine is more common in women suffering from migraine without aura than migraine with aura [27]. The mechanism by which gonadal hormone fluctuations impact migraine frequency is incompletely understood. Somerville was able to postpone migraine attacks in menstrual-migraine sufferers by administration of estradiol, but not by progesterone, suggesting that a drop in estrogen might trigger headache attacks [28]. However, attempts to prevent migraine attacks by continuous estradiol administration were unsuccessful [29].

Oral Contraceptives

Migraine attacks tend to worsen when patients use oral contraceptives (OCPs) [30–32]. The role of these agents as important triggers in migraine is reaffirmed by the finding that women who have headache in association with OCP use have a much lower family history of headache than female migraineurs in general [32]. Bickerstaff reported that many women with common migraine experience a conversion to migraine with aura after taking OCPs [33]. Women with menstrual migraine more frequently report a worsening of their headaches while on OCPs than women with sporadic migraine [34]. If it is assumed that migraine attacks result from withdrawal from high doses of estrogen as implied by Somerville's findings, then attacks should occur during the placebo week of an OCP cycle. This appears to be the case in women with established migraine who have worsening of headache after beginning use of OCPs [31]. However, in women with new onset headaches during use of OCPs, there is not a tendency for the headaches to occur during the placebo week [30, 35]. The fact that a small number of migraineurs show improvement in their headaches after starting OCPs further confuses the issue [36, 37].

It appears that high, stable estrogen levels such as those seen in pregnancy offer some protection against headache, and that abrupt falls in estrogen levels can induce migraine attacks in some women. However, this does not seem to be the only factor or even a consistently over-riding factor in the generation of hormone-associated headaches. Another important consideration for those who decide to begin use of OCPs is that both migraine and OCP use are independent risk factors for stroke in young women [38].

Migraine Headache During Pregnancy

In general, migraine improves during pregnancy [39, 40], although several studies have shown that some women may experience their first migraine attack during pregnancy [41–45]. Migraine that first appears during pregnancy, especially when accompanied by focal neurologic symptoms, is the source of considerable concern and must frequently be distinguished from intracranial hemorrhage, stroke, or sagittal sinus thrombosis. The first trimester is the most common period for new-onset migraine to occur [43]. If migraine occurs during pregnancy, it usually improves during the second and third trimesters [46]. It is not known whether this results from increases in endogenous opiates known to occur during pregnancy, from elevated estrogen levels as suggested above, or from other biochemical alterations that occur during pregnancy.

A large-scale, questionnaire-based study of 400 female headache clinic patients indicated that pregnancy outcomes, breast-feeding rates, and the incidence of hypertension, pre-eclampsia, and eclampsia in migraineurs were similar to those of the general population [47]. However, the risk of female migraineurs developing postpartum depression appeared to be increased [47]. Up to 40% of women experience headache during the first week of the postpartum period. These may be either the TTH or migrainoid headaches. Those experiencing headache are more likely to have had a migraine before pregnancy or a family history of headache [48].

Menopause and Hormone Replacement

Although the conventional wisdom is that migraine attacks cease after menopause, available data seems to support the opposite conclusion. One study found that of 28 postmenopausal migraineurs, 18 had no change in their headache, four were improved or had stopped having headaches, and six were actually worse [49]. Nattero reported that 47% of 1,000 female migraineurs studied had worsening of their migraine after menopause [50]. Epidemiologic data indicates that the female predominance in migraine that begins about the time of menarche reaches a peak female-to-male ratio of 3.3 to 1 between the ages of 40 and 45 and decreases thereafter [2]. However, even after menopause and past the age of 70, the ratio remains at 2 to 1, indicating that cyclic hormonal factors alone cannot fully explain the female predominance [2]. It has been this author's experience that postmenopausal women with persistent headache tend as a group to be fairly refractory to prophylaxis.

The effects of hormone replacement in postmenopausal women are quite unpredictable. Some studies have indicated that administration of estrogen either alone or with progesterone can improve postmenopausal migraine [51–54]. Others have indicated that hormone replacement tends to exacerbate migraine headaches and that a reduction in the dose of estrogen can substantially improve postmenopausal headache [32, 49]. Possible therapeutic maneuvers in patients who require hormone replacement but experience worsening of headaches include reduction of estrogen dose, change from oral to parenteral route, change from animal-derived to synthetic estrogen, or change from interrupted to continuous dosing [55]. Extreme measures such as surgical or medical ovarian ablation for treatment of migraine have proved ineffective [56, 57].

Acute Treatment of Migraine

There is usually some variability in the intensity of migraine attacks. The acute treatment should reflect the severity of the headache. The following agents are appropriate for use in treatment of mild or moderate attacks:

1.   Acetaminophen or NSAIDs, including aspirin, ibuprofen, naproxen and ketoprofen, can be used to treat mild to moderate attacks. Patients should be advised to keep a mild analgesic with them, as prompt treatment can often increase headache-responsiveness to these agents. Pre-emptive treatment with any analgesic should be discouraged, however. Mild to moderate attacks during pregnancy should be treated with acetaminophen. Chronic high-dose use of acetaminophen can lead to liver damage. The main side effects of NSAIDs are gastrointestinal irritation and prolonged bleeding times. Chronic high-dose use of both acetaminophen and NSAIDs has been linked to renal damage.

2.   Midrin, a combination medication containing 325 mg acetaminophen, 65 mg isometheptene mucate (a mild vasoconstrictor), and 100 mg dichloralphenazone (a mild sedative), is frequently effective if taken early in the course of a moderate attack. Two tablets should be taken at the onset of headache followed by one each hour until relief occurs, up to a maximum of five capsules within a 12-hour period. Side effects include dizziness and occasional skin rash.

For treatment of severe attacks, the following agents are recommended:

1.   Fifty milligrams butalbital, a barbiturate, combined with 40 mg caffeine, 325 mg aspirin or 325 mg acetaminophen, or both, in several medications (including Fiorinal, Fioricet, Phrenilin, and Esgic), is one of the most commonly prescribed headache medications. Other preparations add 30 mg codeine. The recommended dosage is two tablets every 4 hours, not to exceed six per day. When used infrequently these medications can be quite effective and are best suited for treatment of moderate to severe infrequent headaches. If used for more than two attacks per month, they can be associated with rebound headaches. Physicians should be vigilant for escalating dose when prescribing this drug. Side effects include dizziness, gastrointestinal disturbance, and sedation.

2.   Oral opiate-containing medications, such as acetaminophen with codeine and oxycodone, have little place in the treatment of chronic, recurrent primary headaches and should be avoided until all other treatment alternatives have been considered. If these medications are the only viable

option due to pregnancy or severe vascular disease, the physician should use them cautiously and discuss risks of rebound headache syndromes and dependency with the patients before prescribing.

3. Ketorolac tromethamine is a NSAID that can be administered intramuscularly (IM) to treat severe migraine attacks with early and severe vomiting. A single preliminary report indicates that it is less effective than dihydroergotamine (DHE) with metoclopramide. Some patients respond well, and in some cases ketorolac may be a viable alternative if intravenous (IV) access is a problem or vasoactive agents, such as DHE or sumatriptan, are contraindicated. Short-term side effects include hypertension, rash, gastrointestinal disturbance, bronchospasm, and increased bleeding time. With long-term chronic use there is a risk of renal damage.

4. Ergotamine, used effectively for many years in the treatment of migraine, is most effective if given early in the migraine attack. It is available in oral, sublingual, and suppository formulations. Overuse of ergotamine can result in a chronic daily headache syndrome and, in extreme cases, the gangrenelike complications of ergotism. Contraindications include coronary artery disease, angina, peripheral vascular disease, Raynaud's phenomenon, uncontrolled hypertension, or severely impaired renal or hepatic function.

5. DHE, an injectable hydrogenated ergot, has less potent peripheral arterial vasoconstrictive effects and can be effective even when given well into the attack. Given by IV, it causes nausea less frequently than ergotamine. However, an antiemetic is usually administered before IV treatment. The following guidelines are provided for the administration of DHE in the acute setting:

- Early in the attack: administer DHE, 1–2 mg IM or subcutaneously. A repeat dose may be given of up to 3 mg in 24 hours.
- Well into a severe attack: administer prochlorperazine, 5 mg IV, or metoclopramide, 10 mg IV, followed in 5–10 minutes by DHE, 0.75–1.00 mg IV given over 2–3 minutes.
- If the attack has not subsided after 30 minutes, an additional 0.5 mg DHE may be given IV.

Side effects of DHE include nausea, vomiting, tingling, transient tachycardia, or bradycardia. The use of metoclopramide or prochlorperazine may sometimes be associated with extrapyramidal side effects. Contraindications are similar to ergotamine tartrate. If the attack persists beyond 72 hours despite treatment (status migrainosus), then repetitive IV doses of DHE are often required. Raskin has established the following protocol for the administration of IV DHE [58].

- Metoclopramide, 10 mg IV, and DHE, 0.5 mg IV, is given over 2–3 minutes.

- If headache stops but nausea develops, no DHE is given for 8 hours, then DHE, 0.3–0.4 mg IV, and metoclopramide, 10 mg IV, is given every 8 hours for 3 days.
- If head pain persists and no nausea develops, DHE, 0.5 mg IV, is repeated in 1 hour; if headache is relieved but nausea develops, DHE, 0.75 mg IV every 8 hours for 3 days with metoclopramide, 10 mg IV, is given; if headache is relieved and no nausea develops, DHE, 1.0 mg IV every 8 hours with metoclopramide, 10 mg IV, is given for 3 days.
- If headache stops and no nausea develops, DHE 0.5 mg IV and metoclopramide, 10 mg IV every 8 hours for 3 days, is administered.

The DHE should be given undiluted through an IV Hep-Lock. Metoclopramide may be discontinued after six DHE doses. Diarrhea is a common side effect of the DHE protocol and can be controlled with oral diphenoxylate. Contraindications to IV DHE include Prinzmetal's angina, pregnancy, coronary artery disease, uncontrolled hypertension, peripheral vascular disease, and severe renal or hepatic disease. Status migrainosus is often associated with overuse of abortive medications and patients should be monitored for evidence of barbiturate or opiate withdrawal.

6. Sumatriptan, a relatively selective serotonergic 5-HT$_{1B/D}$ agonist, exerts both direct vasoconstrictor and antineurogenic inflammatory effects on meningeal vessels. In large-scale, double-blind clinical trials, 6 mg injected subcutaneously significantly reduced headache at 1 hour in over 80% of patients (versus 22% after placebo) [59]. Sumatriptan treatment also reduced the migraine-associated symptoms of nausea, vomiting, photophobia, and phonophobia. It is effective when given up to 4 hours after the onset of a headache attack. Sumatriptan is also available in 25- and 50-mg tablets. Side effects are usually brief and transient and include pressure-like sensations in the head, neck, and chest, tingling in the neck or scalp, and occasional dizziness. Like the ergotamines, sumatriptan is associated with vasoconstriction of coronary arteries. Contraindications include definite or suspected ischemic heart disease, pregnancy, vasospastic angina, or uncontrolled hypertension.

7. Neuroleptics can be an alternative to opiates or vasoactive medications in the treatment of severe migraine attacks in the emergency room setting, although the necessity for an IV and the side effects of hypotension, sedation, and akathisia limit their use. After 500 ml normal saline is administered via IV, chlorpromazine can then be given as a 10-mg IV dose. Frequent blood pressure measurements should be obtained as hypotension is a major side effect. Patients should remain at bed rest for at least an hour after dosing. If the headache persists after 1 hour, the 10-mg dose can be repeated. Alternatively, prochlorperazine, 10 mg IV, can be given without the prior saline infusion and repeated in 30 minutes.

8. Meperidine, an opiate analgesic, is widely administered IM in the emergency room setting to treat severe migraine attacks. With the alterna-

tives now available, the use of parenteral opioids should be limited to patients with very infrequent attacks or patients where other treatments are contraindicated such as severe peripheral or cerebral vascular disease, coronary artery disease, or pregnancy.

Prophylactic Therapy of Migraine

Prophylactic treatment should be considered when attacks occur more than twice per month, are severe enough to prohibit normal activities, or the patient's dread of the attacks limits daily activity. The choice of a prophylactic agent should be based on concomitant illness, other chronic medications, and previous response to medications. Most prophylactic medications were found accidentally to improve migraine. In many cases their effect in migraine is probably unrelated to the action of their original indication. Most prophylactic agents are associated with increased appetite. Patients should be warned about potential weight gain before initiation of treatment.

Prophylactic medications fall into two groups: first-line agents, which are likely to be effective without intolerable side effects, and second-line agents, which may be effective when the first-line agents have failed but are associated with more frequent or potentially serious side effects.

There are four groups of first-line agents: (1) beta-adrenergic blockers, (2) NSAIDs, (3) antidepressants, and (4) calcium channel antagonists. The first group, beta-adrenergic blockers, were originally prescribed as antihypertensive agents. Five beta blockers have been shown in clinical trials to be effective in migraine prophylaxis: propranolol, nadolol, atenolol, timolol and metoprolol [60–65]. These five agents differ in their CNS penetration, their cardioselectivity, and 5-HT binding. Only the lack of partial sympathomimetic activity separates the beta blockers effective in migraine prophylaxis from those that are ineffective. Sometimes patients who do not respond or do not tolerate one beta blocker obtain a good effect with another. Side effects occur in 10–15% of patients and include hypotension, fatigue, depression, dizziness, decreased exercise capacity, gastrointestinal disturbance (diarrhea, constipation), memory disturbance, and insomnia. Contraindications include asthma, congestive heart failure, poorly controlled diabetes, chronic obstructive pulmonary disease, peripheral vascular disease, and cardiac conduction defects.

NSAIDs exert analgesic, anti-inflammatory, and antipyretic effects through their inhibition of cyclooxygenase. Cyclooxygenase inhibition blocks platelet aggregation and the formation of proinflammatory prostaglandins. NSAIDs that have been effective prophylactic agents in controlled clinical trials include aspirin, naproxen, naproxen sodium, tolfenamic acid, ketoprofen, mefenamic acid, and fenoprofen. At present, no clinical trials have compared the efficacy of different NSAIDs. Side effects occurring with chronic use of NSAIDs are similar to those seen with acute use (see the section on Treatment of Migraine: mild to moderate attacks). They are mainly referable to the gastrointestinal tract (dyspepsia, diarrhea, gastritis), but can also include increased bleeding times, and with long-term, high-dose use, renal abnormalities. With toxic levels, tinnitus can occur. Contraindications include peptic ulcer disease, hypersensitivity to other NSAIDs, chronic anticoagulation therapy, renal or liver disease, or age under 12 years. Naproxen sodium is the only agent shown to be effective in the treatment of menstruation-associated migraine in controlled clinical trials [66].

Thus far, the only antidepressant that has shown significant evidence of efficacy in migraine prophylaxis is the tricyclic antidepressant amitriptyline. Other antidepressants sometimes prescribed to treat migraine include fluoxetine, paroxetine, imipramine, clomipramine, and femoxetine. Evidence supporting their use is not well established. Clinical trials also indicate that amitriptyline's antimigraine activity is unrelated to its antidepressant activity [67]. In fact, the doses generally useful in the treatment of migraine are well below those required to treat depression. Amitriptyline may modulate cephalic pain through its inhibition of norepinephrine and serotonin reuptake. Side effects include sedation, dry mouth, photosensitivity of the skin, weight gain, tachycardia, and constipation or urinary retention. Contraindications include narrow-angle glaucoma, pregnancy, urinary retention, and cardiovascular, renal, or liver disease.

The final group of agents used in migraine prophylaxis is the calcium channel antagonists, which block voltage-dependent calcium ionic channels. They are used primarily in the treatment of hypertension. Flunarizine, probably the most effective of these agents in migraine, is not available in the United States. Of those available in the United States, only verapamil has enough evidence of efficacy from double-blind clinical trials to warrant its use. Verapamil has been shown in two small, placebo-controlled, double-blind trials to be superior to placebo in effectiveness [68, 69]. In a third, no significant difference was seen [70]. Although many have found verapamil to be the least effective of the first-line agents, it is sometimes effective when other agents have failed. Therefore verapamil should be tried only when other well-established agents have not been effective or well tolerated. Side effects of verapamil include hypotension, edema, nausea, constipation, and, in some cases, headache. Contraindications include bradycardia, cardiac conduction defects, sick sinus syndrome, and use of beta blockers.

There are three major second-line agents: (1) valproic acid, (2) methysergide, and (3) phenelzine. Valproic acid, an anticonvulsant known to increase endogenous gamma-aminobutyric acid (GABA) levels through its inhibition of GABA aminotransferase and succinate-semialdehyde dehydrogenase, has been shown in several double-blind clinical trials to significantly reduce headache frequency and severity [71–73]. Valproate is the first choice among the second-line agents because of its relatively benign side effect profile at the doses required. It is included as a second-line agent chiefly because it is associated with a 1–2% incidence of neural tube defects in infants born to women taking it during the first trimester of pregnancy. Valproate is the drug of choice for treatment of migraine in patients with bipolar affective disorder. Other side effects include nausea, sedation, tremor, transient hair loss, weight gain, inhibition of platelet aggregation, and minor elevations in liver function tests. Contraindications include hepatic disease, pregnancy, and clotting abnormality.

Methysergide, an ergot derivative, was one of the first drugs used for migraine prophylaxis. Double-blind clinical trials have demonstrated methysergide to be very effective in reducing the frequency, severity, and duration of migraine attacks [74, 75]. Unfortunately, it is associated with the serious complication of retroperitoneal, pericardial, or pleural fibrosis. Because of the risk of this potentially fatal side effect, it should only be used in severe cases that are resistant to the other prophylactic agents. Since the fibrotic complications are reversible early in the process, methysergide should be discontinued for 6–8 weeks every 6 months. The early symptoms of retroperitoneal fibrosis include decreased urine output and leg or back pain. Other potential side effects are nausea, vomiting, depression, sedation, dizziness, lightheadedness, peripheral edema, and vasoconstrictive effects. Contraindications include uncontrolled hypertension, cardiovascular disease, pregnancy, peripheral vascular disease, history of thrombophlebitis or fibrotic disease, and impaired liver or renal function.

Phenelzine, a monoamine oxidase inhibitor, was shown in a single open trial to be effective in 20 of 25 patients with severe migraine [76]. The possibility of the generation of a hypertensive crisis after dietary intake of tyramine-containing foods should limit its use to patients with severe migraine who have been refractory to other treatments and who are committed to strict dietary monitoring. Other side effects include orthostatic hypotension, urinary retention, gastrointestinal disturbance, hepatotoxicity, and failure to ejaculate.

Treatment of Migraine During Pregnancy and Breast-Feeding

The use of all medications during pregnancy and breast-feeding should be reduced as much as possible. See Tables 3.1 and 3.2 for a summary of pregnancy- and lactation-risk categorization of commonly prescribed migraine prophylactic agents and acute headache medications.

During pregnancy, acute treatment should include rest, fluid replacement, and ice packs. Acetaminophen can be used for mild to moderate pain. For more severe pain, oral opiates such as codeine are sometimes used. NSAIDs can be associated with hemorrhagic complications, inhibition of uterine contractions, and narrowing of the ductus arteriosus; they should be avoided in pregnancy. Use of barbiturates and benzodiazepines have been associated in some studies with congenital abnormalities and neonatal withdrawal syndromes and likewise should

TABLE 3.1
Prophylactic Medications Useful in Migraine

Drug	Daily Oral Dose (mg)	Risk to Fetus[a]	Lactation Risk[b]
Beta blockers			
Propranolol (Inderal)	40–240	C	5
Nadolol (Corgard)	20–80	C	5
Atenolol (Tenormin)	50–150	C	5
Timolol (Blocadren)	20–60	C	5
Metoprolol (Lopressor)	50–300	B	5
Nonsteroidal anti-inflammatory drugs			
Naproxen sodium (Aleve, Anaprox)	480–1,100	B[c]	5
Naproxyn (Naprosyn)	750–1,000	B[c]	5
Ketoprofen (Orudis)	150–300	B[c]	5
Aspirin	1,000–1,300	C[c]	4
Antidepressants			
Amitriptyline (Elavil)	10–120	D	3
Ergotamine			
Methylergonovine	0.2–1.0	C	4
Calcium channel blockers			
Verapamil (Calan)	120–480	C	5
Anticonvulsants			
Divalproex sodium (Depakote)	250–1,500	D	5
Serotonin antagonist			
Methysergide (Sansert)	4–8	D	4
Monoamine oxidase inhibitor (Nardil)	30–60	C	3

[a]As determined by the Food and Drug Administration.
[b]As determined by the American Academy of Pediatrics Committee on Drugs.
[c]If drug is taken during third trimester, category is D.
B = no evidence of risk in human beings; C = risk cannot be ruled out; D = positive evidence of human fetal risk; 3 = effects unknown but may be of concern; 4 = use with caution; 5 = usually compatible with breast-feeding.

be avoided [77–79]. The use of ergotamine and DHE is contraindicated in pregnancy. Ergotamine use has been associated with spontaneous abortion, congenital abnormalities such as arrested cerebral development, and jejunal atresia [80, 81].

There are circumstances in which the frequency and severity of attacks and the attendant vomiting can be hazardous to both mother and fetus. In those cases, treatment should first include behavioral modification, relaxation techniques, and avoidance of foods known to trigger attacks. When

TABLE 3.2
Acute Treatments Used in Treating Headache

Drug	Acute Oral Dose (mg)	Risk to Fetus[a]	Lactation Risk[b]
Nonsteroidal anti-inflammatory drugs			
Aspirin	650–975	C	4
Ibuprofen	1,000–1,200	B[c]	5
Naproxen	500–750	B[c]	5
Ketoprofen	50–75	B[c]	5
Acetaminophen	650–1,000	B	5
Ergotamines			
Ergotamine tartrate	0.5–2.0	X	1
Dihydroergotamine	0.5–2.0	X	1
Non-ergot serotonin agonists			
Sumatriptan	25–100	C	3
Opiates			
Codeine	30–60	C[d]	5
Meperidine	50–100	B[d]	5
Morphine	15–30	B[d]	5
Barbiturates		C	
Butalbital	50–100	C	4
Neuroleptics or antiemetics			
Chlorpromazine	10–20	C	3
Prochlorperazine	10–20	C	5
Metoclopramide	10	B	3

[a]As determined by the Food and Drug Administration.
[b]As determined by the American Academy of Pediatrics Committee on Drugs.
[c]If taken during third trimester, category is D.
[d]If taken near term or for prolonged period, category is D.
B = no evidence of risk in human beings; C = risk cannot be ruled out; D = positive evidence of human fetal risk; X = contraindicated in pregnancy; 1 = contraindicated; 3 = effects unknown but may be of concern; 4 = use with caution; 5 = usually compatible with breast-feeding.

these measures have failed, preventative medications may be considered. Use of prophylactic medication during pregnancy should be done cautiously and only with full and informed consent of the patient and her partner. Low-dose propranolol, 10 mg three or four times per day, is sometimes used in these cases; however, no drug can be guaranteed to be safe because most can cross the placenta.

The Food and Drug Administration has five categories of risk for drug use during pregnancy [77–79] (see Tables 3.1 and 3.2):

- Category A: Controlled studies show no risk. Studies in pregnant women show no risk to the fetus.

- Category B: No evidence of risk in human beings. Animal studies show no risk and human studies have not been done, or animal studies have shown adverse effects that were not confirmed in studies in pregnant women.
- Category C: Risk cannot be ruled out. Either adverse effects in animal studies have been present, and there are no human studies, or there are no available animal or human studies. Drug should be used only if potential benefit justifies risk.
- Category D: Positive evidence of human fetal risk. Benefits may possibly justify the risk.
- Category X: Contraindicated in pregnancy. Risk of fetal abnormalities is thought to outweigh any potential benefit.

During breast-feeding, any exposure to a potential toxin via breast milk is probably inappropriate. The concentration of a drug in breast milk is a variable portion of maternal blood level based on several factors, including the drug's molecular weight, ionization, lipophilicity, protein binding, and the presence of active secretion. The infant dose is usually about 1–2% of the maternal dose [82].

The American Academy of Pediatrics Committee on Drugs classifies a medication's risk to the infant during lactation using a 5-point scale [83, 84] (See Tables 3.1 and 3.2). Drugs are categorized as follows:

1. Contraindicated
2. Requires temporary cessation of breast-feeding
3. Effects unknown but may be of concern
4. Use with caution
5. Usually compatible with breast-feeding

Cluster Headache

Cluster headache, the third major primary headache syndrome, is much less common than either migraine or TTH, with a prevalence of about 4 per 1,000 [85]. Cluster headaches afflict men five times as often as women. However, the diagnosis should be considered when a woman presents with severe, unilateral, throbbing or jabbing orbital pain which lasts from 15 minutes to 3 hours. The attacks tend to *cluster*, occurring one or more times daily for a period of weeks or months, then inexplicably going into a remission for months or even years at a time. In an unfortunate few, the clustering pattern may change into a chronic form in which there is no remission. In many patients with the episodic form, headaches assume an uncanny cyclicity, returning at the same time every day. During cluster periods, attacks are often triggered by intake of even small amounts of alcohol or nitrates. The age of onset is typically 20–40 years. Unlike a typical migraine patient, who during a headache seeks to lie quietly in a darkened room, the cluster headache sufferer is often agitated, pacing, and obviously in active distress. The most striking clinical characteristic of the syndrome is the presence of numerous signs of autonomic dysfunction that occur simultaneous with and ipsilateral to the pain. To meet the IHS diagnostic criteria for cluster headache, a patient must have had at least five attacks that consist of severe unilateral orbital or supraorbital and/or temporal pain, which, if untreated, last from 15 to 180 minutes. Attacks are associated with at least one of the following signs ipsilateral to the pain: conjunctival injection, lacrimation, nasal congestion, rhinorrhea, forehead and nasal sweating, miosis, ptosis, and eyelid edema. In addition, they occur with a frequency of at least one attack every other day to eight attacks per day. They are not correlated with any other physical abnormality.

Treatment of Cluster Headache

Almost all cluster headache attacks are severe, so acute treatment is not hierarchic and is geared toward rapid effectiveness.

Oxygen inhalation can be a safe and effective nondrug treatment for acute attacks of cluster headache in many patients. The mechanism of its effect is unknown. Patients most likely to respond to oxygen treatment are those with episodic cluster headaches who are under the age of 50. If this therapy is to be effective, 100% oxygen must delivered at a rate of 8 liters per minute for 15 minutes via a loose-fitting face mask. Nasal cannula administration is usually ineffective. Those who respond to oxygen usually improve within 10 minutes. Unlike vasoconstrictive medications, such as ergotamines and sumatriptan, oxygen is not contraindicated in patients with coronary artery disease or peripheral vascular disease.

Ergotamine tartrate is an effective and well-tolerated treatment in many patients. The sublingual and inhalational routes are superior to oral tablets. DHE may also be of use in the acute treatment of cluster headaches. A double-blind crossover study using intranasal DHE showed an effect on severity of the attacks but no significant effect on the duration [86]. The side effects of ergotamines including nausea and vasoconstriction are described in detail in the section on migraine treatment.

Sumatriptan is effective in reducing both the pain and conjunctival injection of cluster headache within 15 minutes in about three-fourths of patients [87]. It appears to be very well tolerated in cluster headache patients. However, sumatriptan is contraindicated in patients with coronary artery disease, which is quite common among cluster headache sufferers.

Prophylactic Treatment of Cluster Headache

In cluster headache, prophylactic treatment is given only during the cluster period. After a remission is established (usually within 3–6 weeks), the prophylactic agents are tapered and withdrawn.

Verapamil is frequently effective in treating cluster headache at dosages of 240–480 mg per day. One open-labeled trial reported a response rate of 69% in cluster headache [88]. Another double-blind comparison trial found it to be equal to lithium in effect [89].

Ergotamine tartrate is the traditional prophylactic drug of choice in cluster headache. In doses of 2–4 mg per day in either oral or suppository form, ergotamine is an effective, well-tolerated medication for many cluster headache patients [90, 91].

Methysergide is effective in about 70% of cases of episodic cluster headache [92]. Because of the shorter duration of therapy, the development of retroperitoneal, pleural, or pericardial fibrosis, which limits its use in migraine, is much less likely to occur in cluster headache. In cluster headache patients, methysergide should be discontinued for 4–6 weeks after 2–3 months of treatment.

Lithium carbonate has been shown in numerous open clinical trials to be effective in the treatment of chronic cluster headache [93, 94]. It also has beneficial effects in the episodic form. Because of its narrow therapeutic range, serum lithium levels should be monitored throughout the period of treatment. Serum level should be obtained 12 hours after the last dose, should be maintained between 0.3 and 0.8 mmol/liter, and should not exceed 1.0 mmol/liter. Medications such as NSAIDs and thiazide diuretics can cause increases in the serum lithium levels. Average daily doses range from 600 to 900 mg but should be adjusted according to serum concentrations.

Steroids are widely used in the treatment of both the episodic and chronic forms of cluster headache, although evidence of their effect is largely limited to open trials. In a retrospective trial, Couch reported that prednisone (10–80 mg daily) caused marked improvement in 74% of patients [95]. Prednisone in doses of 60–80 mg per day for 1 week followed by a taper over 1–2 weeks is a frequently used protocol. Treatment courses should be brief to avoid side effects such as hyperglycemia, hypertension, psychiatric symptoms, and weight gain.

Chronic Paroxysmal Hemicrania

Chronic paroxysmal hemicrania (CPH) is a relatively rare syndrome of cluster headache that consists of recurrent attacks of severe, clawlike, unilateral orbital-temporal pain [96]. It has an estimated prevalence of about 3%. CPH is similar to cluster headache in that the attacks are associated with various autonomic signs ipsilateral to the head pain, including conjunctival injection, lacrimation, nasal congestion, rhinorrhea, ptosis, and eyelid edema [13]. It differs from cluster headache in several respects. Females are affected more frequently than males, with a 7-to-3 female-to-male ratio. The attacks tend to be very brief (2–25 minutes) and occur more frequently (more than five per day for more than half of the time). The maximal frequency is in excess of 25 attacks per day. Prolonged remissions usually do not occur, although some patients seem to pass through a nonchronic stage during which remissions can occur. Attacks are very responsive to indomethacin (150 mg or less per day). However, attacks often return upon tapering of the medication, suggesting that it is only a symptomatic treatment.

Attacks of CPH can be triggered by bending or rotating head movements [96] as well as by external pressure on the transverse processes of C4–C5, the C2 root, or the greater occipital nerve [97]. The female predominance and reports of remission during pregnancy have suggested a hormonal influence [98].

Treatment of CPH with indomethacin, in an initial dose of 25 mg twice a day, is titrated upward over several days until the attacks cease (sometimes requiring up to 150–250 mg per day). After relief is stable for several days, the dose should be lowered to the minimum effective maintenance dose (usually 25–100 mg daily). There is great interindividual variation in the maintenance dose required. Indomethacin can have serious gastrointestinal side effects when given chronically. These include dyspepsia, peptic ulcer, and gastrointestinal bleeding. Other potential side effects include dizziness, nausea, and purpura.

Secondary Headache with Female Predominance

Benign Intracranial Hypertension

Benign intracranial hypertension (BIH), or pseudotumor cerebri, is a relatively common neurologic disorder (estimated annual incidence of from 0.9 to 1.7 per 100,000) [99, 100]. It occurs in all age groups. There is no female predominance in children. However, in adults the female-to-male ratio is from 3 to 10 to 1 [99, 101, 102]. It is most common in overweight women of childbearing age (annual incidence 19 per 100,000) [99]. In BIH, increased intracranial pressure occurs in the absence of hydrocephalus or intracranial mass. The resulting syndrome is characterized by headache, papilledema, transient visual blurring, normal cerebrospinal fluid (CSF) composition, and absence of local neurologic signs.

The diagnosis is made by lumbar puncture (CSF pressure greater than 250 mm H_2O; normal CSF composition) after neuroimaging has excluded a mass lesion. An enlarged blind spot is often found on visual-field testing. Visual fields and acuity should be monitored periodically. Spontaneous recovery is characteristic, but therapy geared toward prevention of vision loss is usually instituted.

Treatment of Benign Intracranial Hypertension

Medical treatment with acetazolamide (250–1,000 mg per day) to decrease CSF production is the first line of treatment. Other diuretics such as furosemide or thiazides are also sometimes effective. Repeated lumbar punctures are sometimes used to lower CSF pressure. However, with the frequent side effect of post–lumbar puncture headache, this method is seldom agreeable to patients. Weight loss can be an effective treatment and should be recommended to most patients. However, sustained weight loss in this patient population can be difficult. In patients who do not respond to medical therapy or who show evidence of vision loss, surgical intervention in the form of ventricular-peritoneal or lumbar-peritoneal shunting procedures is indicated [103]. Alternatively, optic nerve fenestration can be used to treat the papilledema and protect against vision loss. Oddly, unilateral fenestration is reported to relieve papilledema in both eyes [103]. The headaches of BIH can persist despite reversal of papilledema and normalization of CSF pressures. In these instances, migraine drugs such as propranolol and naproxen can be helpful [103].

Conclusion

Women are disproportionately afflicted with headaches, a common source of suffering and disability in Western society. Chronic TTH, migraine, CPH, and pseudotumor cerebri all commonly affect young women during years of peak professional productivity and childrearing. The reasons for female predominance in these syndromes is incompletely understood. Many women experience remission during the last 6 months of pregnancy when stable hormone levels are present, suggesting that hormone fluctuation might be an important factor in headache generation among women. Treatment of headache syndromes should be based on careful, accurate clinical diagnosis and may require preventive as well as acute medications. The use of medication during pregnancy and breast-feeding should be minimized as much as possible. As the demands of coping with both employment and family responsibilities continue to increase, the suffering inflicted on women by these disorders is likely to increase as well. The continued investigation of both the pathophysiologic basis and the mechanisms of the hormonal involvement in these syndromes is critical to the development of safer and more effective treatments for headaches in women.

References

1. Taylor H (ed). The Nuprin Report. New York: Louis Harris & Associates, 1985.
2. Stewart WF, Lipton R, Celantano DD, et al. Prevalence of migraine headache in the United States. JAMA 1992;267:64.
3. Ray BS, Wolff HG. Experimental studies on headache. Pain-sensitive structures of the head and their significance in headache. Arch Surg 1940;41:813.

4. Mayberg MR, Zervas NT, Moskowitz MA. Trigeminal projections to supratentorial pial and dural blood vessels in cats demonstrated by horseradish peroxidase histochemistry. J Comp Neurol 1984;223:46.

5. Moskowitz MA. Neurogenic inflammation in the pathophysiology and treatment of migraine. Neurology 1993;43(Suppl 3):S16.

6. Celantano DD, Linet MS, Stewart WF. Gender differences in the experience of headache. Soc Sci Med 1990;30:1289.

7. Nikiforow R. Headache in a random sample of 200 persons: a clinical study of a population in northern Finland. Cephalalgia 1981;1:99.

8. Rasmussen BK, Jensen R, Schroll M, et al. Epidemiology of headache in a general population—a prevalence study. J Clin Epidemiol 1991;44:1147.

9. Crisp AH, Kalucy RS, McGuinness B, et al. Some clinical, social and psychological characteristics of migraine subjects in the general population. Postgrad Med J 1977;53:691.

10. Waters WE, O'Connor PJ. Epidemiology of headache and migraine in women. J Neurol Neurosurg Psychiatr 1971;34:148.

11. Friedman AP, von Storch TJC, Merritt HH. Migraine and tension headaches: a clinical study of two thousand cases. Neurology 1954;4:773.

12. Rasmussen BK. Migraine and tension-type headache in a general population: psychosocial factors. Int J Epidemiol 1992;21:1138.

13. Olesen J (ed). IHS classification and diagnostic criteria for headache disorders, cranial neuralgias and facial pain. Cephalalgia 1988;8(Suppl 7):9.

14. Diamond S, Baltes BJ. Chronic tension-type headache treated with amitriptyline: a double-blind study. Headache 1971;11:110.

15. Fogelholm R, Murros K. Maprotiline in chronic tension headache: a double-blind cross-over study. Headache 1985;25:273.

16. Morland TJ, Storli OV, Mogstad TE. Doxepin in the prophylactic treatment of mixed vascular and tension headache. Headache 1979;19:382.

17. Bussone G, Sandrini G, Ruiz L, et al. Effectiveness of Fluoxetine on Pain and Depression in Chronic Headache Disorders. In G Nappi, G Bono, G Sandrini, et al. (eds), Headache and Depression: Serotonin Pathways as a Common Clue. New York: Raven, 1991;265.

18. Bickerstaff ER. Basilar artery migraine. Lancet 1961;1:15.

19. Sturzenegger MH, Meienber O. Basilar artery migraine: a follow-up study of 82 cases. Headache 1985;25:408.

20. Joutel A, Bousser MG, Biousse V, et al. Migraine hemiplegique familiale localization d'un gene responsible sur le chomosome 19. Rev Neurol 1994;150:340.

21. Bille B. Migraine in school children. Acta Paediatrica 1962;51(Suppl 136):1.

22. Grant ECG. Relation of arterioles in the endometrium to headache from oral contraceptive. Lancet 1965;1:1143.

23. Diamond S, Dalessio DJ. The Practicing Physician's Approach to Headache. Baltimore: Williams & Wilkins, 1982.

24. Lance J, Anthony M. Some clinical aspects of migraine. A prospective survey of 500 patients. Arch Neurol 1966;15:356.

25. Digre K, Damasio H. Menstrual migraine: differential diagnosis, evaluation and treatment. Clin Obstet Gynecol 1987;30:417.
26. Epstein MT, Hockaday JM, Hockaday TDR. Migraine and reproductive hormones throughout the menstrual cycle. Lancet 1975;1:543.
27. Cupini LM, Matteis M, Troisi E, et al. Sex-hormone-related events in migrainous females. A clinical comparative study between migraine with aura and migraine without aura. Cephalalgia 1995;15:140.
28. Somerville BW. The role of estradiol withdrawal in the etiology of menstrual migraine. Neurology 1972;22:355.
29. Somerville BW. Estrogen-withdrawl migraine II. Attempted prophylaxis by continuous estradiol administration. Neurology 1975;25:245.
30. Phillips BM. Oral contraceptive drugs and migraine. BMJ 1968;2:99.
31. Whitty CWM, Hockaday JM, Whitty MM. The effect of oral contraceptives on migraine. Lancet 1966;1:856.
32. Kudrow L. The relationship of headache frequency to hormonal use in migraine. Headache 1975;15:36.
33. Bickerstaff ER. Neurological complications of oral contraceptives. Oxford: Clarendon Press, 1975.
34. Dalton K. Migraine and oral contraceptives. Headache 1975;15:247.
35. Welch KMA, Darnley D, Simkins RJ. The role of estrogen in migraine: a review and hypothesis. Cephalalgia 1968; 4:227.
36. Larson-Cohn U, Lundberg PO. Headache and treatment with oral contraceptives. Acta Neurol Scand 1970;46:267.
37. Edelson RN. Menstrual migraine and other hormonal aspects of migraine. Headache 1985;25:376.
38. Lindegaard O. Oral contraceptives, pregnancy and the risk of cerebral thromboembolism: the influence of diabetes, hypertension, migraine and previous thrombotic disease. Br J Obstet Gynecol 1995;102:153.
39. Critchley M, Ferguson FR. Migraine. Lancet 1933;1:123.
40. Lance JW, Anthony M. Some clinical aspects of migraine. Arch Neurol 1966;15:356.
41. Ratinahirana H, Darbois T, Bousser MG. Migraine and pregnancy: a prospective study in 702 women after delivery. Neurology 1990;40(Suppl 1):437.
42. Callaghan N. The migraine syndrome in pregnancy. Neurology 1968;18:197.
43. Somerville BWA. Study of migraine in pregnancy. Neurology 1972;22:824.
44. Wright GDS, Patel MK. Focal migraine and pregnancy. BMJ 1986;293:1557.
45. Chancellor AM, Wroe SJ, Cull RE. Migraine occurring for the first time in pregnancy. Headache 1990;30:224.
46. Noronha A. Neurologic disorders during pregnancy and the puerperium. Clin Perinatol 1985;12:706.
47. Loder E. Pregnancy in migraineurs: medication use, outcomes, and complications. Abstract presented at the American Association for the Study of Headache Scientific Meeting, June 2, 1996, San Diego, CA.
48. Stein G, Morton J, Marsh A, et al. Headaches after childbirth. Acta Neurol Scand 1984;69:74.

49. Whitty CW, Hockaday JM. Migraine: a follow-up study of 92 patients. BMJ 1968;1:735.
50. Nattero G. Menstrual headache. Adv Neurol 1982;33:215.
51. Campbell S. Double-Blind Psychometric Studies on the Effects of Natural Estrogens on Postmenopausal Women. In S Campbell (ed), The Management of the Menopause and Postmenopausal Years. Baltimore: University Park Press, 1975;149.
52. Martin PL, Burnier AM, Segre EJ, et al. Graded sequential therapy in the menopause: a double blind study. Am J Obstet Gynecol 1971;111:178.
53. Dennerstein L, Morse C, Burrows G, et al. Menstrual migraine: a double blind trial of percutaneous estradiol. Gynecol Endocrinol 1988;2:113.
54. Greenblatt RB, Bruneteau DW. Menopausal headache—psychogenic or metabolic. J Am Geriatr Soc 1974;283:186.
55. Silberstein SD, Merriam GR. Estrogens, progestins and headache. Neurology 1991;41:786.
56. Utian WH. Oestrogen, headache and oral contraceptives. S Afr Med J 1974;48:2105.
57. Alvarez WC. Can one cure migraine in women by inducing menopause? Mayo Clin Proc 1940;380.
58. Raskin NH. Repetitive intravenous dihydroergotamine as therapy for intractable migraine. Neurology 1986;36:995.
59. Moskowitz MA, Cutrer FM. Sumatriptan: a receptor targeted treatment for migraine. Annu Rev Med 1993;44:145.
60. Weber RB, Reinmuth OM. The treatment of migraine with propranolol. Neurology 1972;22:366.
61. Ryan RE Sr, Ryan RE Jr, Sudilovsky A. Nadolol: its use in the prophylactic treatment of migraine. Headache 1983;23:26.
62. Johannsson V, Nilsson LR, Widelius T, et al. Atenolol in migraine prophylaxis: a double-blind cross-over multicenter study. Headache 1987;27:372.
63. Forssman B, Lindblad,CJ, Zbornikova V. Atenolol for migraine prophylaxis. Headache 1983;23:188.
64. Stellar S, Ahrens SP, Meibohm AR, et al. Migraine prevention with timolol. JAMA 1984;252:2576.
65. Kangasneimi P, Hedman C. Metoprolol and propranolol in the prophylactic treatment of classical and common migraine: a double-blind study. Cephalalgia 1984;4:91.
66. Sargent J, Solbach P, Damasio H, et al. A comparison of naproxen sodium to propranolol hydrochloride and a placebo control for the prophylaxis of migraine headaches. Headache 1985;25:320.
67. Couch JR, Hassanein RS. Amitriptyline in migraine prophylaxis. Arch Neurol 1979;36:695.
68. Solomon GD, Steel JG, Spaccavento LJ. Verapamil prophylaxis of migraine: a double-blind placebo-controlled trial. JAMA 1983;250:200.
69. Markley H, Cheronix J, Piepho R. Verapamil prophylactic therapy of migraine. Neurology 1984;34:973.

70. Solomon GD, Scott AFB. Verapamil and propranolol in migraine prophylaxis: a double blind crossover study. Headache 1986;26:325.
71. Hering R, Kuritzky A. Sodium valproate in the prophylactic treatment of migraine: a double-blind study versus placebo. Cephalalgia 1992;12:81.
72. Jensen R, Brinck T, Oleson J. Sodium valproate has a prophylactic effect in migraine without aura: a triple-blind, placebo-crossover study. Neurology 1994;44:647.
73. Coria F, Sempere AP, Duarte J, et al. Low-dose sodium valproate in the prophylaxis of migraine. Clin Neuropharmacol 1994;17:569.
74. Pedersen E, Moller CE. Methysergide in migraine prophylaxis. Clin Pharmacol Therap 1966;7:520.
75. Southwell N, Williams JD, Mackenzie I. Methysergide in the prophylaxis of migraine. Lancet 964;1:523.
76. Anthony M, Lance JW. Monoamine oxidase inhibition in the treatment of migraine. Arch Neurol 1969; 21:263.
77. Briggs GG, Freeman RK, Yaffe SJ. Drugs in Pregnancy and Lactation (3rd ed). Baltimore: Williams & Wilkins, 1990.
78. Niebyl JR, Lietman PS. The Use of Mild Analgesics in Pregnancy. In JR Niebyl (ed), Drug Use in Pregnancy (2nd ed). Phildelphia: Lea & Febiger, 1988;21.
79. Silberstein S. Headache and women: treatment of the pregnant and lactating migraineur. Headache 1993;33:533.
80. Hughes HE, Goldstein DA. Birth defects following maternal exposure to ergotamine, beta blockers and caffeine. J Med Genet 1988;25:396.
81. Graham JM, Marin-Padilla M, Hoefnagel D. Jejunal atresia associated with Cafergot ingestion during pregnancy. Clin Pediatr 1982;22:226.
82. Niebyl JR. Teratology and Drugs in Pregnancy and Lactation. In R Winters (ed), Danforth's Obstetrics and Gynecology (6th ed). Philadelphia: Lippincott, 1990.
83. American Academy of Pediatrics Committee on Drugs. The transfer of drugs and other chemicals into human breast milk. Pediatrics 1983;72:375.
84. American Academy of Pediatrics Committee on Drugs. The transfer of drugs and other chemicals into human breast milk. Pediatrics 1989;84:924.
85. Heyck H. "Cluster"-Kopfschmerz (Bing-Horton-Syndrome). Fortschr Neurol Psychiatr Grenzgeb 1976;44:37.
86. Anderssen PG, Jespersen LT. Dihydroergotamine nasal spray in the treatment of attacks of cluster headache. Cephalalgia 1986;6:51.
87. The Sumatriptan Cluster Headache Study Group. Treatment of acute cluster headache with sumatriptan. N Engl J Med 1991;325:322.
88. Gabai IJ, Spierings ELH. Prophylactic treatment of cluster headache with verapamil. Headache 1989;29:167.
89. Bussone G, Leone M, Peccarisi C, et al. Double blind comparison study of lithium and verapamil in cluster headache prophylaxis. Headache 1990;30:411.
90. Ekbom KA. Ergotamine tartrate orally in Horton's "histaminic cephalalgia" (also called Harris's "ciliary neuralgia"). Acta Psychiatr Scand 1947;46(Suppl):106.

91. Horton BT. Histaminic cephalalgia. Lancet 1952;2:92.
92. Curran DA, Hinterberger H, Lance JW. Methysergide. Res Clin Stud Headache 1967;1:74.
93. Kudrow L. Lithium prophylaxis for chronic cluster headache. Headache 1977;17:15.
94. Mathew NT. Clinical subtypes of cluster headache and response to lithium therapy. Headache 1978;18:26.
95. Couch JR, Ziegler DK. Prednisone therapy for cluster headche. Headache 1978;18:219.
96. Antonaci F, Sjaastad O. Chronic paroxysmal hemicrania (CPH): a review of the clinical manifestations. Headache 1989;29:648.
97. Sjaastad O, Russell D, Saunte C, et al. Chronic paroxysmal hemicrania. 6. Precipitation of attacks. Further studies on the precipitation mechanism. Cephalalgia 1982;2:211.
98. Stein HJ, Rogado AZ. Chronic paroxysmal hemicrania: two new patients. Headache 1980;20:72.
99. Durcan FJ, Corbett JJ, Wall M. The incidence of pseudotumor cerebri. Population studies in Iowa and Louisiana. Arch Neurol 1988;45:875.
100. Radhakrishnan K, Sridharan R, Ashok PP, et al. Pseudotumor cerebri: incidence and pattern in North-Eastern Libya. Eur Neurol 1986;25:117.
101. Corbett JJ. The 1982 Silversides Lecture. Problems in the diagnosis and treatment of pseudotumor cerebri. Can J Neurol Sci 1983;10:221.
102. Wall M. Idiopathic intracranial hypertension. A prospective study of 50 patients. Brain 1991;114:155.
103. Sorensen PS, Corbett JJ. High Cerebrospinal Fluid Pressure. In J Olesen, P Tfelt-Hansen, KMA Welch (eds), The Headaches. New York: Raven, 1993;679.

CHAPTER 4

Neuro-Oncologic Diseases

Tracy Batchelor

Neuro-oncologic diseases include both primary and metastatic tumors of the nervous system as well as nonmetastatic disorders such as paraneoplastic complications. Some neuro-oncologic diseases occur more commonly or exclusively in women.

Primary Brain Tumors

Epidemiology

Approximately 17,500 people in the United States will be diagnosed with a primary brain tumor this year, and 11,000 will die from this disease [1, 2]. Incidence rates of nearly all primary brain tumors are higher in males of all ages and geographic regions [2, 3]. The age-adjusted sex ratios (male to female) for specific histologic types of brain tumors are 1.69 for oligodendroglioma, 1.61 for glioblastoma multiforme, 1.45 for astrocytoma, and 1.03 for malignant meningioma [2]. However, surveillance data on meningiomas have consistently shown higher incidence figures in females with a sex ratio of 0.6 in one study. Pituitary adenomas are also more common in females across all age groups [2, 3].

Meningiomas

Meningiomas are tumors that are thought to arise from meningothelial cells that make up the arachnoid villi of the meninges [4]. These lesions account for approximately 20% of all intracranial and 25% of all intraspinal tumors. The incidence of these tumors increases with age [5, 6].

The incidence of meningiomas is approximately twice as high in women as in men [7]. Specifically, intracranial meningiomas are twice as common and intraspinal meningiomas nine times as common in women

[5]. Meningiomas also seem to have a relationship with sex hormones; accelerated growth of these tumors occurs during the luteal phase of the menstrual cycle and during pregnancy [7, 8]. There may also be an increased incidence of meningiomas in women with breast cancer, although one study contests this relationship [9–11]. Many studies have examined the role of androgen, estrogen, and progesterone receptors in meningiomas. Most found progesterone and androgen receptors in a high proportion of meningioma specimens and low levels of estrogen receptors in a small proportion of specimens, which were obtained at the time of initial surgery and at recurrence. Other reports suggest there may be aberrant estrogen receptors present that escape detection by conventional methods [7, 8, 12, 13]. Progesterone receptors have been found, on average, in 72% of meningiomas with a range of 28–98%. The wide range may be accounted for in part by the different sensitivities of the analytic methods used to measure progesterone receptors [14, 15]. The progesterone receptors are thought to be functionally important and may have a role in the regulation of meningioma growth [5, 8]. A small number of studies have suggested that the presence of progesterone receptors in meningiomas correlates with less aggressive clinical behavior as well as histologic type, with meningothelial and transitional meningiomas more often positive for the presence of progesterone receptors than are fibrous meningiomas [14, 16, 17]. However, most studies have found no clear relationship between progesterone-receptor activity and age, sex, histologic type, tumor size, clinical behavior, and menstrual status [8]. Androgen receptors have also been found in a high percentage of meningiomas, and there may be a correlation between these receptors and progesterone receptors in meningiomas [7].

The association of meningiomas with sex steroids provides an opportunity for use of hormonal therapy in treating these tumors. The progesterone-receptor antagonist mifepristone (RU 486) has been studied as a potential antitumor agent in meningiomas. Mifepristone has been shown to inhibit the growth of meningioma cell lines in vitro and exerts a growth-inhibitory effect on human meningiomas transplanted into mice [18, 19]. Although there have been a limited number of human studies, preliminary results are encouraging. One study using neuroimaging found that six of 10 patients with progressive meningiomas showed stabilization or slight regression of the tumors during treatment for 12 months with mifepristone, 200 mg per day. There was no information on the receptor status of these tumors and there were significant side effects, including nausea, vomiting, and fatigue, all of which are attributable to the glucocorticoid-blocking effect of mifepristone [18]. Another study of 14 patients showed objective tumor regression on computed tomography (CT) or magnetic resonance imaging (MRI) in 35% of individuals treated with this agent [20]. Studies of the antiestrogen-agent tamoxifen have demonstrated less activity, perhaps due to the low frequency of estrogen receptors in meningiomas. Partial responses were observed in one of six cases and in one of nine cases [12]. Further trials with antiandrogen agents and more specific antiprogesterone agents with less glucocorticoid-blocking activity are indicated based on these preliminary results.

Despite the promise of hormonal therapy of meningiomas, surgery remains the mainstay of treatment. Although it is believed by many that surgery for meningiomas is curative and safe, operative mortality rates as high as 14% have been reported and 10-year survival rates vary from 43% to 77%. Even with gross total removal, 10-year recurrence rates of 9–20% have been reported; with subtotal resection these figures increase to 18–50%. Adjunctive radiation therapy has been shown to increase local control rate, time to recurrence, and survival for subtotally resected lesions [8].

Since most in vivo studies do not demonstrate a clear relationship between the presence of progesterone receptors and tumor size or behavior, interruption of hormone therapy in postmenopausal women with small or asymptomatic meningiomas does not seem warranted as long as these individuals can be followed closely with careful clinical and radiographic evaluations [14].

Pituitary Tumors

Pituitary tumors account for approximately 15% of all primary intracranial neoplasms and occur with higher frequency in women, particularly during the child-bearing years. The female preponderance of these tumors is due to the increased frequency of prolactinomas in women in the second and third decades of life. Women are affected four times more often than men and account for 78% of all those with prolactinomas (Figure 4.1) [21].

Pituitary tumors arising from the glandular tissue are termed *adenomas* and are arbitrarily divided on the basis of size into microadenomas (<10 mm) and macroadenomas (>10 mm). These may present clinically with a finding of endocrine dysfunction or displacement of surrounding structures such as the optic chiasm or pain-sensitive dura. Pituitary adenomas can result in excess secretion of any anterior pituitary hormone. The most common clinical syndromes resulting from excess pituitary hormones are amenorrhea-galactorrhea (excess prolactin), acromegaly (excess growth hormone), and Cushing's disease (excess adrenocorticotrophic hormone). Other hormone-secreting adenomas are rare.

Prolactinomas result in a clinical syndrome of infertility; amenorrhea or irregular menses; and a thin, milky-white discharge from the nipples, which occurs either spontaneously or with stimulation (amenorrhea-galactorrhea syndrome) [22]. Hyperprolactinemia results in a relative or absolute estrogen deficiency that may cause accelerated osteopenia and predispose an individual to later osteoporosis [23]. Because of these clinically apparent

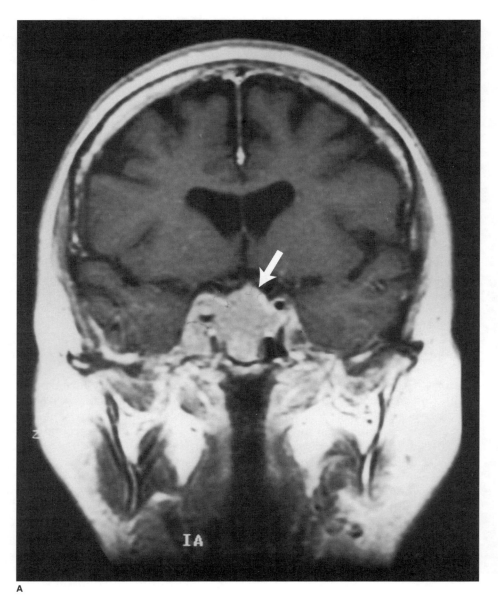

A

FIGURE 4.1. Coronal (A) and sagittal (B) T1-weighted, gadolinium-enhanced cranial magnetic resonance images of a homogenously enhancing, prolactin-secreting macroadenoma (*arrows*) with expansion of the sella and invasion of surrounding structures.

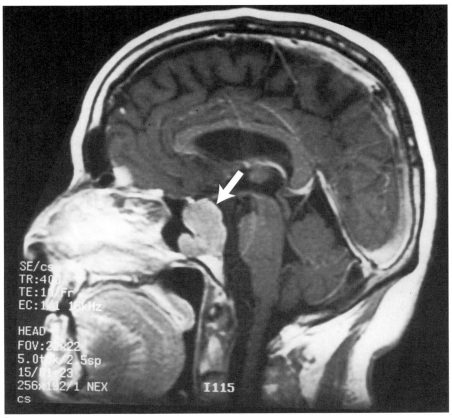

B

symptoms, prolactinomas in women are usually discovered while the tumor is still small (<1 cm); in men, however, prolactinomas are often not found until a later stage of growth. These tumors produce an elevation of the serum prolactin level usually in excess of 150 ng/ml. However, because the secretion of prolactin from the anterior lobe of the pituitary is under the inhibitory control of dopamine from the hypothalamus, any disruption in the transport of this substance through the hypophyseal portal system results in elevation of serum prolactin. This is termed the *stalk-section effect* and may be produced by any pituitary mass and result in hyperprolactinemia, even though the elevation is usually in the range of 30–100 ng/ml, below the level typically observed with prolactinomas [24].

Medical therapy of prolactinomas is possible with the dopamine-agonist bromocriptine, a potent inhibitor of the synthesis and release of prolactin by the pituitary gland. This drug has no tumoricidal activity; instead, it decreases the size of the tumor by decreasing cytosolic volume [25]. Subsequent withdrawal of bromocriptine may result in re-expansion of the tumor and return of hyperprolactinemia, although at least one study suggests this is uncommon [24, 26]. Whether the preoperative use of bromocriptine enhances the rate of surgical cure remains controversial [24, 27]. Long-term use (greater than 1 year) of the drug may increase fibrosis within the tumor and thus reduce the possibility of surgical cure [28]. Bromocriptine is likely to be a good option in patients with a low chance of surgical cure due to prolactin levels in excess of 500 ng/ml [29].

Surgery remains the mainstay of treatment for most pituitary tumors; transsphenoidal microsurgery provides the most direct and rapid approach to the tumor. According to one authority, the indications for surgery of prolactin-secreting macroadenomas include clinical evidence of mass effect (vision loss), apoplexy, resistance to bromocriptine, and desire for fertility [30]. The surgical cure rate for macroadenomas is approximately 50%, with the best surgical candidates having prolactin levels of less than 200 ng/ml [21]. Although the best surgical results are obtained with prolactin-secreting microadenomas, management remains controversial. In young women who want to become pregnant, surgery is probably the best option because many physicians do not recommend use of bromocriptine during pregnancy and there is also a risk of accelerated tumor growth during pregnancy [31, 32]. Curative tumor resection and subsequent pregnancy has been achieved in 84% of such patients [21, 33]. In women with moderate elevations of prolactin who do not plan to become pregnant, conservative management with serial clinical examinations, serum prolactin levels, and MRI studies or medical treatment with bromocriptine are options. Given the usual success of medical and surgical treatment of prolactinomas, radiation therapy has a limited role in their management, although one small series has achieved durable reduction in prolactin levels and tumor size with irradiation [27, 34].

Effects of Pregnancy

The incidence of all cancer during pregnancy is estimated to be in the range of 0.07% to 0.1% [35]. Approximately one in 44,000 pregnancies is complicated by the diagnosis of a maternal brain tumor with approximately 89 cases identified in the United States each year [36]. There were 223 reported cases of a primary brain or spinal cord tumor diagnosed during pregnancy as of 1987 [37]. However, the incidence of primary brain tumors that become symptomatic in pregnant women 15–44 years old is lower than expected for this age group [37, 38]. Similarly, the age at first pregnancy and the number of pregnancies do not appear to affect brain tumor risk [39]. The reason the incidence of brain tumors in pregnancy is lower than expected is not known, although women with subclinical cancer may become pregnant less often or experience disruption of their pregnancies more frequently [38]. The relative frequency of different primary brain tumor types is not changed by pregnancy, with 85% of such tumors consisting of meningiomas, gliomas, pituitary tumors, and vestibular schwannomas. However, basal meningiomas and vascular spinal tumors are more common in pregnancy [37, 40]. Most of these tumors are diagnosed during the first pregnancy and are most likely to become symptomatic in the third trimester. However, gliomas tend to accumulate in the first trimester with the onset of meningiomas increasing during the second and third trimesters. Although the relative frequency of meningiomas and prolactinomas does not appear to increase in relation to pregnancy, tumor progression and symptoms do increase over this period. The reason for this tumor growth in pregnancy is not clearly known; however, some authorities have suggested it is due to engorgement of blood vessels or expansion of the intracellular fluid space, while others contend hormonal influences may be involved [36]. A review found 44 cases of maternal cancer had metastasized to the products of conception, with 12 such cases involving the fetus. In the latter cases the maternal cancer was either a lymphoproliferative neoplasm or a melanoma [35, 36].

Since the symptoms of increased intracranial pressure (ICP) (headache upon awakening, nausea, and vomiting) are similar to the symptoms of morning sickness, evaluation can be challenging [40]. Should neuroimaging of the pregnant patient with these symptoms become necessary, MRI is the procedure of choice because there is no exposure to ionizing radiation [36]. Although there is no evidence that MRI affects the fetus, this imaging modality should be avoided if possible in the first trimester because exposure to powerful electromagnetic fields occurs [41]. Similarly, there is very little data regarding the safety of the ferromagnetic contrast agent gadolinium, which is not sanctioned for use during pregnancy and should be avoided if possible [40]. In the patient with rapid neurologic deterioration, CT may be necessary. This does involve radiation exposure of approximately 2.5–3.0 rad to the head of the patient and a fetal exposure estimated to be 1 mrad or less per slice. Fetal exposure can be reduced by appropriate shielding of the uterus with a lead apron [35]. With fetal exposures less than 10 rad, no adverse effects occur in excess of the background rate of spontaneous abnormalities in 3% of live births and the spontaneous abortion rate of 30% in all pregnancies [35, 40]. Medically indicated exposures of up to 5 rad are considered acceptable in pregnancy when unavoidable. There has been limited experience with the use of iodinated contrast agents during pregnancy, and the risks are not precisely defined. Such agents should be avoided in the first trimester [40].

Treatment of brain tumors or their complications may be necessary during pregnancy. Cerebral edema and increased ICP may require the use of glucocorticoids and mannitol. Glucocorticoids have been used during pregnancy for other reasons, including the prevention of neonatal respiratory distress syndrome. There is no evidence of resultant growth, physical, motor, or developmental deficiencies within the first 3 years of life [42]. However, fetal adrenal suppression may occur with long-term, high-dose therapy during any part of pregnancy and necessitates the use of supplemental steroids in the peripartum period [43]. Although mannitol does cross the placenta and is excreted by the fetal kidney into the amniotic fluid, no adverse effects have been reported with its use [44, 45].

Cranial irradiation exposes the fetus to higher doses of radiation than diagnostic imaging. In general, radiation exposure in utero carries a risk of adverse fetal outcomes including spontaneous abortion, anatomic malformation, growth and mental retardation, and possibly childhood cancer. The risk of childhood cancer is highest with exposure during the first trimester [35, 40]. The exposure to the fetus from scatter is less when conventional radiation therapy is delivered to parts distant from the uterus; such exposure carries low risk. Strategies to reduce fetal exposure include the use of focal rather than whole-brain irradiation, radiation dose reduction, substitution of heavy charged particles for photons, and deferring radiation until after delivery [40].

Chemotherapy typically involves agents that are teratogenic in the first trimester and associated with adverse fetal outcomes [35]. Properties of chemotherapeutic agents that improve permeability across the blood-brain barrier also facilitate transport across the placenta, making these drugs especially hazardous. Although there are data to suggest that certain chemotherapeutic agents are associated with minimal risk in the second and third trimesters, chemotherapy for malignant brain tumors should be avoided during pregnancy [35, 40].

The method of delivery to be used for a pregnant woman with a brain tumor remains controversial. Perhaps the most important factor is the presence and severity of increased ICP. During labor, uterine contractions do not typically increase ICP in the mother, although abdominal pressure in the second stage of labor does significantly elevate ICP [36]. One authority has suggested that the decision of whether to perform a cesarean section should be based on obstetric reasons alone and that if there is unusual concern about intracranial hypertension, a forceps delivery is indicated to avoid the second stage of labor [36]. However, cesarean section is usually recommended in the presence of increased ICP, although other maternal and fetal factors such as parity, neurologic condition of the mother, location and grade of tumor, and position and health of the fetus are important in making this decision [40].

Effects of Menopause

Menopause is associated with a decline and eventual cessation of estrogen synthesis and a relative increase in the synthesis of progesterone and androgens. Women who have undergone natural menopause seem to have a reduced risk for development of meningiomas, which may be attributable to this decline in estrogen levels. In women who have undergone bilateral oophorectomy (artificial menopause), there is complete and immediate cessation of ovarian hormone production, which confers not only a reduced risk for meningiomas but for other brain tumors as well, implicating these hormones in tumor growth. Bilateral oophorectomy after natural menopause does not further reduce the risk of brain tumors [39].

Neurologic Complications of Cancer

Breast Cancer

Breast cancer is the most common malignancy among women in North America, accounting for 27% of all cancers. Approximately 181,000 new cases of breast cancer were diagnosed in 1992, and 46,000 women died from the disease the same year [46]. Neurologic complications occur in approximately 25% of patients with metastatic breast cancer although autopsy studies have demonstrated central nervous system (CNS) involvement in 31–57% of examinations [46–48].

Cranial Metastases

Metastases from breast cancer may involve the skull, dura, or brain. Skull metastases are common and are usually associated with disease in other bones. Calvarial metastases may cause localized headache or swelling but are usually asymptomatic. Metastases to the base of skull are less common but are more likely to produce symptoms or signs from compression of cranial nerves [49]. Metastases to the mandible may involve the mental nerve and produce the "numb chin syndrome," which includes unilateral numbness of the lower lip, chin, and mucous membranes on the inside of the lip. Such lesions are usually visible on CT or plain radiographs of the mandible and treatment with regional radiation results in symptomatic improvement in most patients [50]. Breast cancer is the most common cause of dural metastases, which are found on autopsy to affect 16–18% of patients with breast cancer [47, 51]. These are often asymptomatic but may cause symptoms by compression or invasion of brain, cranial nerves, or venous sinuses. These dural lesions may resemble meningiomas on neuroimaging studies, and since there may be an increased frequency of meningiomas in breast cancer patients, they can cause diagnostic confusion [48].

Breast cancer is the leading cause of brain metastases in women and is estimated to be responsible for 10–20% of such cases [47, 52]. At the time of diagnosis these lesions are single in 56–58% of cases and multiple in 42–44% of cases [48, 53]. Brain metastases develop more frequently and earlier in the course of the disease in premenopausal women; however, menopausal status does not affect survival [48, 54]. One study found that a brain metastasis was the first site of relapse in 20% of cases, although most brain metastases occur in the context of progressive extracranial disease [55]. The most frequent presenting symptoms include new seizure, subacute onset of headache, altered mentation, or gait disturbance [48]. The most sensitive diagnostic study is a gadolinium-enhanced cranial MRI (Figure 4.2). Treatment options include steroids, radiation, surgery, or chemotherapy. Dexamethasone, 16 mg per day, will result in symptomatic improvement in 70–80% of patients with brain metastases [56]. Whole-brain irradiation and steroids result in improvement or stabilization of symptoms in 95% of patients [48, 52]. Follow-up cranial CT scans demonstrate disappearance and regression of lesions in 35% and 40% of patients, respectively. However, median survival with this approach is only 3–4 months, with 21% of patients surviving beyond 1 year [52]. All patients who are to receive whole-brain irradiation should be maintained on steroids for 48–72 hours before initiation of radiation to reduce intracranial pressure and minimize acute radiation toxicity [56]. In patients without extensive extracranial disease, single, surgically accessible brain metastases can be excised with improvement in survival rates and quality of life [57]. Studies have suggested that stereotactic radiosurgical approaches achieve results similar to resection for single or multiple brain metastases [58]. Chemotherapy has not been a conventional approach for brain metastases, although there is emerging interest in the treatment of brain metastases from breast cancer with this modality. Studies using a number of drug combinations have demonstrated response rates and median survival times comparable to whole-brain irradiation [52, 55, 59, 60]. Because approximately 50% of breast cancer patients with brain metastases will die of progressive extracranial disease, the ultimate prognosis for the majority of these patients depends on the control of disease outside the brain. A possible advantage of systemic chemotherapy is the ability to treat both the intracranial and extracranial sites of disease simultaneously [52]. However, chemotherapy has not been compared to radiation for this population in a prospective randomized clinical trial.

Other intracranial sites of metastases in breast cancer patients include the optic nerve and pituitary gland. Although optic nerve metastases are rare, breast cancer is the most common cause of such lesions. Presentation is a usually painless and slowly progressive unilateral vision loss with optic disc edema on examination. Metastasis to the choroid occurs in approximately 10% of cases of advanced breast cancer and presents with decreased visual acuity with scotoma. Symptomatic visual impairment should be treated with irradiation. Pituitary metastases from breast cancer have been demonstrated in 9% of cases at autopsy. Most of these lesions are asymptomatic but may cause headache, ophthalmoplegia, or diabetes insipidus. Vision loss and hypopituitarism are uncommon symptoms and more suggestive of a pituitary adenoma if there is no other evidence of metastasis [48].

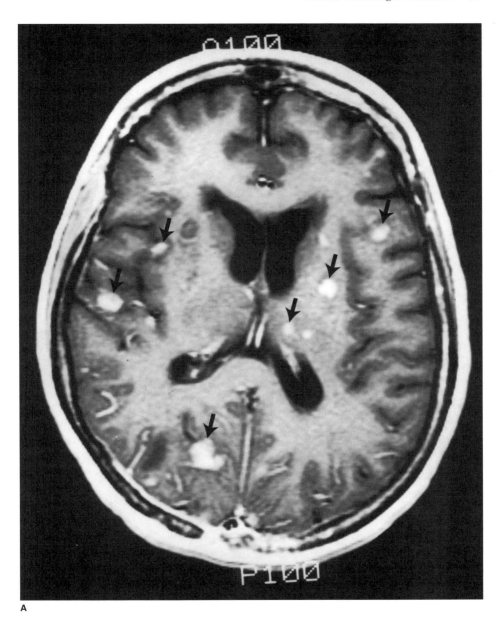

A

FIGURE 4.2. A. Axial T1-weighted, gadolinium-enhanced cranial magnetic resonance image of a woman with breast cancer demonstrating multiple, enhancing brain metastases (*arrows*).

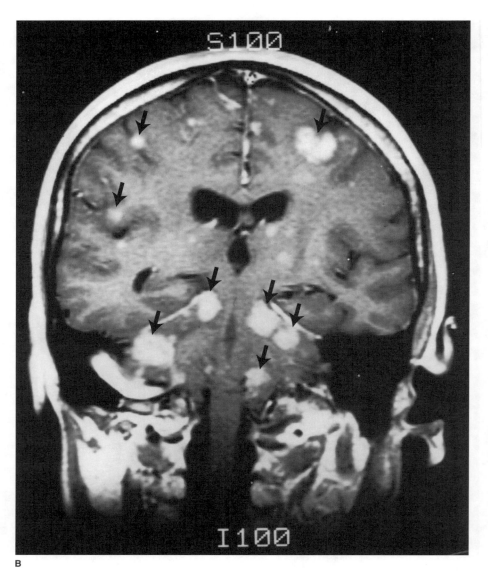

B

FIGURE 4.2.   B. Coronal T1-weighted, gadolinium-enhanced cranial magnetic resonance image of the same patient.

Leptomeningeal Metastases

Leptomeningeal metastases (LM) from breast cancer occur in 2–5% of patients with metastatic disease, although some studies suggest that only half of such cases are diagnosed during life [48, 61]. Breast cancer is the most common cause of LM and accounts for 50% of cases associated with solid tumors [62]. LM can occur at any time during the course of breast cancer, and clinical presentation is usually subacute with multifocal symptoms and signs reflecting involvement of multiple levels of the neuraxis (brain, cranial nerves, and spinal roots) [63, 64]. In addition to cranial nerve palsies, which occur in 80% of cases of LM, altered mentation, headache, meningismus, seizures, and gait disturbance also occur in varying frequencies. Diagnostic evaluation should include cerebrospinal fluid (CSF) analysis, which typically shows a mononuclear pleocytosis with elevated protein and low glucose levels. Identification of malignant cells in the CSF is diagnostic [65]. However, since this is a qualitative test with significant interobserver variability, multiple samples are usually necessary [61]. Autopsy studies of patients with LM demonstrate that approximately 50% have a positive cytology after a single lumbar puncture (LP), with an additional 30% discovered after a second LP [64, 65]. In addition, cisternal puncture increased the yield of positive cytologies by 25% in one study of solid tumors with LM [61]. Interest in CSF tumor markers may result in better diagnostic capability in the future [61]. Neuroimaging of the brain with CT or MRI may demonstrate effacement of the sulci and cisterns, ependymal or cortical nodule enhancement, hydrocephalus, or normal imaging. Spinal imaging with MRI or myelography may show nodular or diffuse thickening of nerve roots or CSF block, which occurs in approximately 70% of LM cases associated with solid tumors and is an important prognostic factor [66, 67]. Despite poor prognosis and poor response to treatment in LM associated with most solid tumors, the breast cancer subset of LM is more amenable to treatment. Treatment usually includes delivery of intrathecal chemotherapy via dural puncture or indwelling-ventricular reservoir [62]. Multiple drug therapy does not seem to confer an advantage over single-agent treatment with methotrexate [68]. In patients with focal symptoms or CSF block, localized spinal radiation is a treatment option. Median survival with treatment is 6–8 months, with 15–25% of such patients surviving more than 1 year [62, 64].

Treatment with intrathecal methotrexate may result in acute meningoencephalitis with confusion, headache, fever, nausea, and vomiting approximately 2–4 hours after the injection. Pleocytosis and elevated protein levels are usually seen on CSF evaluation. Symptoms usually resolve over 12–72 hours but may recur with subsequent treatments. Myelopathy and sudden death are rare complications of intrathecal methotrexate [48].

Approximately 50% of breast cancer patients who survive more than 1 year with LM metastases treated with repeated injections of intrathecal methotrexate develop a leukoencephalopathy that includes confusion, dementia, somnolence, or focal neurologic signs [62]. This usually occurs when intrathecal methotrexate is combined with whole-brain irradiation, and this combination should be avoided if possible. The leukoencephalopathy may improve if intrathecal methotrexate is discontinued, although it may also progress to coma and death [48].

Epidural Metastases

Epidural spinal cord compression (ESCC) occurs in 3–4% of patients with breast cancer during life, with a 5–10% frequency at autopsy [69]. In cancer hospitals breast cancer is the leading cause of ESCC, accounting for 22% of all cases [48]. ESCC is most commonly the result of direct spread of the tumor from the bony elements of the spine to the epidural space. Vertebral body metastases occur in 60% of patients with breast cancer and may be the consequence of mammary vein drainage into the vertebral venous plexus. Compression of nerve roots or spinal cord may result from spread of tumor into the epidural space or intervertebral foramina or by collapse of the vertebral body with encroachment of tumor and bone into the epidural space [48]. ESCC from breast cancer involves the thoracic spine in 75–80% of cases, cervical spine in 15%, and lumbosacral spine in 6–7% [70]. Compression of the spine at more than one level is not uncommon and mandates evaluation of the entire spine. The most common presenting symptom is pain that is usually confined to the back but may become radicular with progression. Weakness and sensory loss may follow, with bladder and bowel symptoms usually occurring later. In one retrospective study of symptoms in 70 breast cancer patients with ESCC, 96% had motor weakness, 94% pain, 79% sensory disturbance, and 61% sphincter disturbance [69]. Progression usually occurs over weeks to months, but sudden deterioration may occur in 20% of patients [71]. Urgent investigation is mandated if ESCC is suspected.

Women in complete remission from breast cancer are unlikely to present with ESCC as first relapse (only two of 70 cases in one study) [69]. The majority of women presenting with ESCC have existing bone metastases (93% in study); therefore, this group of women should be evaluated urgently. Although plain x-rays are abnormal at the symptomatic level in 94% of patients with breast cancer and ESCC, spinal MRI is the preferred diagnostic test to identify ESCC (Figure 4.3). When other modalities are used initially, most patients eventually undergo a series of progressively advanced diagnostic tests to identify ESCC [72]. One advantage of MRI is the ability to image the entire neuraxis, thus identifying any areas of asymptomatic disease. If back pain precludes the ability of the patient to cooperate for the prolonged time necessary for MRI, then myelography should be performed. In patients with neurologic signs of ESCC, steroids should be started before spinal imaging. Animal studies and anecdotal experience suggest high-dose dexamethasone is beneficial in patients with spinal cord compression. In patients with severe pain or myelopathy, treatment with dexamethasone, 100-mg intravenous (IV) bolus followed by 24 mg IV every 6 hours, is recommended with tapering of the drug after more definitive therapy has been started. In patients without neurologic signs, 16 mg per day in four divided doses is recommended [72]. Definitive treatment of ESCC

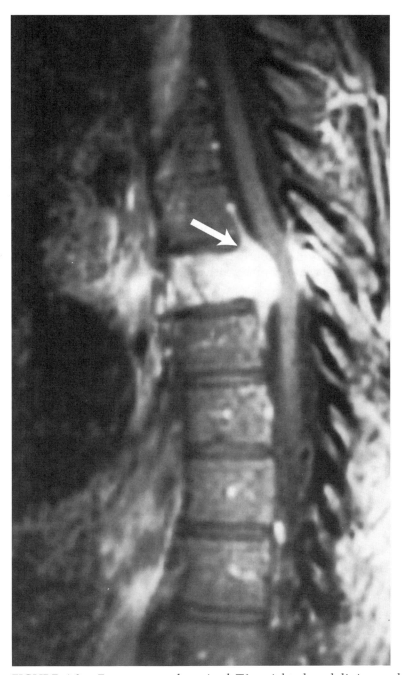

FIGURE 4.3. Fat-suppressed, sagittal T1-weighted, gadolinium-enhanced spinal magnetic resonance image demonstrating enhancement of a thoracic vertebral body with an associated epidural metastasis (*arrow*) compressing the spinal cord.

consists of radiation therapy or surgery. The goals of therapy are pain alleviation and maintenance or return of neurologic function. Most studies have failed to demonstrate a difference in outcome between radiation alone versus surgery followed by radiation [69]. Most authorities recommend initiation of radiation therapy immediately after identification of involved spinal levels on MRI or myelography [72]. Surgery may have a role in patients who have been previously irradiated, in patients who progress despite radiation, or in cases with spinal instability. Ambulatory status at presentation is the most important factor predictive of neurologic outcome, thus emphasizing the need for rapid evaluation and diagnosis [73, 74]. In one study, all ambulatory patients at the start of radiation could walk post-treatment, while 74% of paraparetic patients and 33% (one of three) of paraplegic patients regained the ability to walk [74]. The ability to ambulate is also strongly associated with improved survival in breast cancer patients with ESCC. In general, prognosis is poor in cancer patients with ESCC, with only 30% surviving more than 1 year in one study. However, the breast cancer subset of patients with ESCC has a better prognosis, with 29% of patients surviving more than 3 years in this same study [74].

Intramedullary spinal metastases are rare but breast cancer accounts for 15% of all cases. Many of these patients will also have brain metastases. Presentation is usually with back pain and progressive asymmetric myelopathy. Diagnosis is best made by MRI; treatment with steroids and radiation may improve neurologic function [48].

Neuromuscular Complications

Malignant infiltration of the brachial plexus occurs in approximately 2.5% of all women with breast cancer [48]. The tumor usually compresses or invades the plexus from below with neurologic symptoms progressing from lower to upper plexus. Severe pain in the shoulder and arm usually precedes other symptoms by weeks to months. The sensory symptoms are usually followed by progressive weakness and wasting beginning in the small muscles of the hand and progressively involving more proximal parts of the arm. Horner's syndrome may result if the tumor extends into the paraspinal or epidural space. Other signs include induration and tenderness in the supraclavicular fossa, lymphedema of the arm, and trophic changes in the skin and nails [48, 72].

Evaluation of the brachial plexus includes electromyography (EMG), which may show neurogenic changes including fibrillations, and nerve conduction studies, which may demonstrate prolonged or absent F waves and lowered sensory and compound motor action potentials. Imaging of this region includes CT and MRI, which may show a mass or loss of normal tissue planes. Imaging should include evaluation of the epidural space with MRI or myelography if such extension is suspected. However, a normal imaging study does not exclude malignant infiltration of the brachial plexus and surgical exploration may be necessary [48].

The brachial plexus may be involved by other processes in women with breast cancer, and these should be included in the differential diagnosis. In women who have received radiation to the axilla or upper thorax (after mastectomy for breast cancer), several complications may arise. An acute brachial plexitis with mild pain and shoulder weakness can begin approximately 4 months after local radiation therapy for breast cancer. Although the weakness may be severe, it is usually reversible. Radiation fibrosis usually occurs in 2–4% of patients after radiation, although frequencies as high as 15% have been reported. It tends to develop more than 6 months after completion of radiation and is usually painless, with involvement of the muscles of the shoulder before the hand. Horner's syndrome is uncommon, but lymphedema is more common than in cases of malignant infiltration of the plexus. Myokymia on EMG is considered pathognomonic of radiation fibrosis. The T2-weighted signal on MRI of the brachial plexus tends to be low in radiation fibrosis and high in cases of malignant infiltration. A late complication of radiation is occlusion of the subclavian artery, which can result in sudden development of weakness without pain. Angiography may be necessary to demonstrate the occlusion [48, 72].

The treatment of malignant infiltration of the brachial plexus by breast cancer is radiation. This can reduce the size of the tumor and may partially relieve the pain. However, relief is usually incomplete and further treatment with narcotic analgesics, nerve blocks, and cordotomy may be necessary.

Involvement of the lumbosacral plexus by metastatic breast cancer is uncommon, usually occurring in the context of sacral and pelvic bone metastases. Slowly progressive pain in the back, buttock, and thigh are early symptoms, with later development of unilateral asymmetric lymphedema, weakness, and loss of sensation and reflexes in the involved leg. Evaluation includes rectal examination since the mass may be palpable, as well as EMG and nerve conduction studies, which usually show neurogenic muscle changes and decreased amplitudes of sensory and motor action potentials, respectively. Imaging with CT or MRI usually reveals bone metastases, adenopathy, and a mass in the region of the plexus. The treatment is the same as for malignant infiltration of the brachial plexus [48].

Approximately 4–6% of postmastectomy patients will develop pain due to injury to the intercostobrachial nerve or cutaneous branches of the intercostal nerves. A constricting or burning sensation in the axilla, posteromedial upper arm, and anterior chest wall is the usual complaint. Onset may be immediate or delayed for up to 6 months after surgery. Treatment includes tricyclic antidepressants, nerve blocks, and topical anesthetics [75–77].

Paraneoplastic Complications

The paraneoplastic complications most commonly occurring in breast cancer are cerebellar degeneration and the anti-Ri syndrome.

Paraneoplastic cerebellar degeneration typically begins with slight incoordination while walking, with progression over weeks to months to an incapacitated state. The symptoms and signs are usually pancerebellar with both appendicular and truncal ataxia; however, approximately 50% of patients will have other neurologic signs on examination. The cerebellar symptoms precede the identification of the cancer in approximately two-thirds of patients. Evaluation may include a lumbar puncture, which usually shows a lymphocytic pleocytosis, elevated protein levels, IgG, and positive oligoclonal bands in the early phases of the illness. The cranial CT and MRI studies are often normal early in the illness but may show diffuse cerebellar atrophy later in the course. Most patients with paraneoplastic cerebellar degeneration in the context of breast cancer have serum antibodies (anti-Yo) that react against the cytoplasm of Purkinje cells [72]. Although the disease is thought to be immune-mediated, therapies such as plasmapheresis and immunosuppressants have been disappointing in these patients [78]. Reports of anecdotal success with immunoadsorption therapy require further study [79].

Breast cancer has been identified in six of 11 reported cases of the anti-Ri syndrome. The symptoms of opsoclonus, myoclonus, and truncal ataxia typically wax and wane, with some patients experiencing spontaneous resolution. There is usually a CSF pleocytosis and elevation of protein, although cranial CT and MRI are usually normal [72, 80]. By definition, all of these patients have an antineuronal antibody (anti-Ri) that is similar to the anti-Hu antibody that reacts with the nuclei of virtually all neurons of the central and peripheral nervous system. Since there have been so few cases and there is waxing and waning of symptoms, efficacy of specific treatments is not known.

Stiff-man syndrome is a rare neurologic disorder characterized by fluctuating muscular rigidity and spasms and the presence of antibodies against glutamic acid decarboxylase in the majority of patients. Five cases of paraneoplastic stiff-man syndrome have been reported, including three with adenocarcinoma of the breast. All of the breast cancer cases had an antibody against a 128-kd neuronal protein. Detection of this antibody in any patient with stiff-man syndrome should prompt a search for an occult breast cancer [81].

Other Neurologic Complications

Intracranial hemorrhages from brain metastases are unusual in breast cancer patients, although thrombocytopenia from chemotherapy, radiation, or bone marrow metastasis may result in intracerebral or subdural hemorrhages. Dural metastases may result in subdural bleeding, and radiation should follow surgery if such disease is identified at that time. Breast cancer is one of the most common causes of disseminated intravascular coagulation in cancer patients and may result in small cerebral infarctions from multiple fibrin thrombi, producing confusion and focal neurologic signs. Approximately 5–10% of cases of nonbacterial thrombotic endocarditis occur in women with breast cancer. Platelet/fibrin vegetations form on the heart valves, resulting in cardiogenic cerebral embolism and infarcts. Cranial CT or MRI will demonstrate such infarcts, and angiography may show multiple embolic occlusions. IV heparin may be beneficial [72].

Metabolic disorders may produce potentially reversible behavioral changes in breast cancer patients; hypercalcemia is one of the more common causes of such behavioral changes. Complications of breast cancer therapy include methotrexate leukoencephalopathy and radiation injury of the brachial plexus, as previously described. Tamoxifen may produce a retinopathy that can impair vision; however, vision may improve after discontinuation [48].

Gynecologic Cancers

Ovarian Cancer

Ovarian cancer does not usually involve the nervous system. However, with improved treatment for ovarian cancer, longer survival may increase the frequency of such complications.

Brain metastasis is a rare complication of ovarian cancer, with only 67 well-documented cases in the literature, according to one review. A multi-institutional study of 4,027 ovarian cancer patients over 30 years identified only 32 cases, while an autopsy study of ovarian cancer reported an incidence of 0.9% [82, 83]. However, there is some evidence that this complication may be increasing, with studies reporting brain metastases in 1–4% of such patients [83]. Serous cystadenocarcinoma is the most common histology associated with brain metastases [84]. The clinical presentation is similar to other solid tumors, with brain metastases occurring an average of 14.5 months after diagnosis of the ovarian tumor [85]. Approximately 50–90% of women with brain metastases from ovarian cancer will have extra- or intraperitoneal disease at the time of diagnosis. Conventional treatment has consisted of dexamethasone and whole-brain irradiation. Most patients treated in this manner achieve palliation until death. Median survival in the multi-institutional study of 32 patients was 4 months with whole-brain irradiation, while other studies report survival times from 3 to 10 months [82]. The addition of surgical resection, stereotactic radiosurgery, and chemotherapy may improve these results [83, 84].

LM metastasis is also a rare complication of ovarian cancer, with only 14 cases reported by 1994. The presentation is similar to LM metastasis from other solid tumors. In the single case in which it was measured, CSF CA-125 was elevated [86]. Treatment is usually with intrathecal methotrexate, radiation, or both. Response rates vary among the few cases reported.

According to one authority, ovarian cancer is the second leading cause of the approximately 300 reported cases of paraneoplastic cerebellar degeneration [72]. A subset of patients with ovarian cancer will have antibodies in the serum and CSF directed against the cytoplasm of Purkinje cells (anti-Yo) [88]. The presence of the anti-Yo antibody should prompt evaluation of the breast and reproductive organs. One authority has suggested that failure to identify a cancer on routine gynecologic examination, mammography, and pelvic CT should lead to examination under general anesthesia followed by a dilatation and curettage. Finally, hysterectomy and bilateral salpingo-oophorectomy should be considered in those remaining women with no identifiable gynecologic pathology. With few exceptions, therapies such as plasmapheresis and immunosuppression do not appreciably alter the disease course [72, 78, 87].

Neurologic complications may result from chemotherapy directed against ovarian cancer. Paclitaxel and docetaxel are novel chemotherapeutic agents that promote polymerization and inhibit depolymerization of microtubules. They are commonly used in patients with ovarian cancer [89]. Approximately 60% of patients receiving a paclitaxel dose of 250 mg/m^2 develop paresthesias of the hands and feet. Although in most patients the symptoms do not progress and may improve, this toxicity may be dose-limiting. Arthralgias and myalgias in the legs can develop 2–3 days after treatment with these drugs and may last for 2–4 days. A distal sensory and sensorimotor neuropathy as well as a neuropathic proximal motor weakness may also complicate treatment with these drugs [89]. One report demonstrates that the neuropathy is axonal in nature [90]. Nerve-growth factor prevents paclitaxel neuropathy experimentally, and clinical trials are underway using this agent. Paclitaxel has also been associated with a reversible encephalopathy in a small number of reports [91].

Cisplatin changes the cell cycle by binding covalently to DNA bases. The drug is effective against ovarian cancer and may be combined with paclitaxel in some protocols. Peripheral neuropathy is the most common neurotoxicity of cisplatin and is common in doses greater than 400 mg/m^2. The neuropathy, which involves large-fiber sensory axons, begins in the toes and feet with progression to more proximal areas of the arms and legs. Proprioceptive loss may produce sensory ataxia and impair gait. Treatment is ineffective after the neuropathy has started, although the neuropathy usually improves if the patient survives the cancer. Lhermitte's sign may appear during or shortly after treatment with cisplatin and presumably represents a transient demyelinating lesion in the posterior columns of the spinal cord. Ototoxicity may result from cisplatin damage of hair cells and is usually subclinical, involving the high-frequency range. Acute deafness has been reported with high-dose cisplatin. Vestibular toxicity is less common than hearing loss and involves vertigo, oscillopsia, and nausea. Seizures, cortical blindness, and encephalopathy very rarely follow IV cisplatin [72, 92].

Cervical Cancer

A review of 121 cases of invasive cervical cancer demonstrated epidural spinal cord compression in five cases, with two cases occurring at initial diagnosis of cervical cancer. Back pain is not an unusual complaint in many patients with cervical cancer and has been attributed to the presence of the pelvic tumor. However, this report suggests consideration of epidural metastasis is important as early diagnosis and treatment may prevent neurologic deterioration. The prognosis remains poor with a median survival of 4 months in this series [93].

Choriocarcinoma/Gestational Trophoblastic Disease

Choriocarcinoma is a rare tumor of the placenta with an incidence of approximately one in 50,000 term pregnancies and one in 30 molar pregnancies [94, 95]. Brain metastases occur in 10–20% of patients with choriocarcinoma, and two-thirds of patients who die with this disease have brain metastases [85, 96]. Intratumoral hemorrhage is not uncommon with this type of brain metastasis. Human chorionic gonadotropin (hCG) is a sensitive tumor marker produced by gestational trophoblastic neoplasms and may be elevated in both the serum and CSF when brain metastases are present. The level of hCG is commonly followed serially as a measure of treatment effectiveness [94]. Although mortality from choriocarcinoma is higher in those patients with brain metastases, the overall prognosis is more favorable than in patients with brain metastases from other primary tumors, with an approximately 80–90% chance of long-term survival after chemotherapy and whole-brain irradiation [96]. One established approach includes systemic methotrexate, actinomycin D, and chlorambucil with intrathecal methotrexate and whole-brain irradiation of up to 3,000 cGy over 10 fractions [85]. Serum and CSF hCG should be within the normal range for at least 12 months before discontinuing such therapy. Neoplastic intracranial aneurysms may occur when an embolic tumor lodges in an intracerebral vessel and invades the vessel wall. Rupture of such an aneurysm may produce subarachnoid or intracerebral hemorrhage. This complication usually occurs in advanced cases of choriocarcinoma and may be associated with cardiac metastases [85, 96].

Conclusion

Neuro-oncologic diseases of women involve tumors that arise within the CNS and the neurologic complications of tumors that originate outside the nervous system. Although all primary brain tumors may occur in both sexes, meningiomas and pituitary tumors occur with greater frequency in women and may be influenced by hormonal factors. Sex steroids affect tumor growth and may provide an opportunity for the development of hormonal therapies. The unique hormonal and vascular changes of pregnancy may also affect tumor size and management. Fetal development and the physical changes of pregnancy complicate the management of brain tumors during this period. Breast cancer is the most common type of cancer in women and results in more neuro-oncologic complications than perhaps all other tumors combined. Neurologic management of these complications requires knowledge of the specific metastatic and non-metastatic conditions associated with this disease.

References

1. Lesser GJ, Grossman S. The chemotherapy of high-grade astrocytomas. Semin Oncol 1994;21:220.
2. Radhakrishnan K, Bohnen NI, Kurland LT. Epidemiology of Brain Tumors. In RA Morantz, JW Walsh (eds), Brain Tumors. New York: Marcel Dekker, 1994;1.
3. Giles GG, Gonzalez MF. Epidemiology of Brain Tumors and Factors in Prognosis. In AH Kaye, ER Laws (eds), Brain Tumors. New York: Churchill Livingstone, 1995;47.
4. Young B. Surgery of Benign Brain Tumors. In RA Morantz, JW Walsh (eds), Brain Tumors. New York: Marcel Dekker, 1994;429.
5. Carroll RS, Glowacka D, Dashner K, et al. Progesterone receptor expression in meningiomas. Cancer Res 1993;53:1312.
6. DeMonte F, Al-Mefty O. Meningiomas. In AH Kaye, ER Laws (eds), Brain Tumors. New York: Churchill Livingstone, 1995;675.
7. Carroll RS, Zhang J, Dashner K, et al. Androgen receptor expression in meningiomas. J Neurosurg 1995;82:453.
8. Black PM. Meningiomas. Neurosurgery 1993;32:643.
9. Rubinstein AB, Schein M, Reichenthal E. The association of carcinoma of the breast with meningioma. Surg Gynecol Obstet 1989;169:334.
10. Schoenberg BS, Christine BW, Whisnant J. Nervous system neoplasms and primary malignancies of other sites. Neurology 1975;25:705.
11. Jacobs DH, Holmes FF, McFarlane MJ. Meningiomas are not significantly associated with breast cancer. Arch Neurol 1992;49:753.
12. Rubinstein AB, Loren D, Geier A, et al. Hormone receptors in initially excised versus recurrent intracranial meningiomas. J Neurosurg 1994;81:184.
13. Koehorst SGA, Jacobs HM, Tilanus MGJ, et al. Aberrant estrogen receptor species in human meningioma tissue. J Steroid Biochem Mol Biol 1992;43:57.
14. Bouillot P, Pellissier J-F, Devictor B, et al. Quantitative imaging of estrogen and progesterone receptors, estrogen-regulated protein, and growth fraction:

immunocytochemical assays in 52 meningiomas. Correlation with clinical and morphological data. J Neurosurg 1994;81:765.

15. Piantelli M, Pinelli A, Macri E, et al. Type II estrogen binding sites and anti-proliferative activity of quercetin in human meningiomas. Cancer 1993;71:193.

16. Lesch KP, Grass S. Estrogen receptor immunoreactivity in meningiomas. Comparison with the binding activity of estrogen, progesterone, and androgen receptors. J Neurosurg 1987;67:237.

17. Markwalder TM, Zara DT, Goldhirsch A, et al. Estrogen and progesterone receptors in meningiomas in relation to clinical and pathologic features. Surg Neurol 1983;20:42.

18. Lamberts SWJ, Tangha HLJ, Arezaat CJJ, et al. Mifepristone (RU 486) treatment of meningiomas. J Neurol Neurosurg Psychiatry 1992;55:486.

19. Maxwell M, Galanopoulos T, Neville-Golden J, et al. Expression of androgen and progesterone receptors in primary human meningiomas. J Neurosurg 1993;78:456.

20. Grunberg SM, Weiss MH, Spitz IM, et al. Treatment of unresectable meningiomas with the anti-progesterone agent mifepristone. J Neurosurg 1991;74:861.

21. Thapar K, Laws ER. Pituitary Tumors. In AH Kaye, ER Laws (eds), Brain Tumors. New York: Churchill Livingstone, 1995;759.

22. Forbes AP, Henneman PH, Griswold GC, et al. Syndrome characterized by galactorrhea, amenorrhea and low urinary FSH: comparison with acromegaly and normal lactation. J Clin Endocrinol Metab 1954;14:265.

23. Klibanski A, Neer RM, Beitins IZ, et al. Decreased bone density in hyperprolactinemic women. N Engl J Med 1980;303:1511.

24. Barrow DL, Tindall GT. Tumors of the Pituitary Gland. In RA Morantz, JW Walsh (eds), Brain Tumors. New York: Marcel Dekker, 1994;367.

25. McGregor AM, Scanlon MF, Hall K, et al. Reduction in size of a pituitary tumor by bromocriptine therapy. N Engl J Med 1979;300:291.

26. van't Verlaat JW, Croughs RJM. Withdrawal of bromocriptine after long-term therapy for macroprolactinomas; effect on plasma prolactin and tumor size. Clin Endocrinol 1991;34:175.

27. Klibanski A, Zervas NT. Diagnosis and management of hormone-secreting pituitary adenomas. N Engl J Med 1991;324:822.

28. Landolt AM, Keller PJ, Froesch ER, et al. Bromocriptine: does it jeopardise the result of later surgery for prolactinomas? Lancet 1982;2:657.

29. Barrow DL, Mizuno J, Tindall GT. Management of prolactinomas associated with very high serum prolactin levels. J Neurosurg 1988;68:554.

30. Randall RV, Laws ER, Abboud CF, et al. Transphenoidal microsurgical treatment of prolactin-producing pituitary adenomas. Results in 100 patients. Mayo Clin Proc 1983;58:108.

31. Gonzalez JG, Elizondo G, Saldivar D, et al. Pituitary gland growth during normal pregnancy: an *in vivo* study using magnetic resonance imaging. Am J Med 1988;85:217.

32. Kupersmith MJ, Rosenberg C, Kleinberg D. Visual loss in pregnant women with pituitary adenomas. Ann Intern Med 1994;121:473.
33. Laws ER, Fode NC, Randall RV, et al. Pregnancy following transphenoidal resection of prolactin-secreting pituitary tumors. J Neurosurg 1983;58:685.
34. Mehta AE, Reyes FI, Faiman C. Primary radiotherapy of prolactinomas. Am J Med 1987;83:49.
35. Doll DC, Ringenberg S, Yarbro JW. Management of cancer during pregnancy. Arch Intern Med 1988;148:2058.
36. Simon RH. Brain tumors in pregnancy. Semin Neurol 1988;8:214.
37. Roelvink NCA, Kamphorst W, van Alphen HAM, et al. Pregnancy-related primary brain and spinal tumors. Arch Neurol 1987;44:209.
38. Haas JF, Janisch W, Staneczek W. Newly diagnosed primary intracranial neoplasms in pregnant women: a population-based assessment. J Neurol Neurosurg Psychiatry 1986;49:874.
39. Schlehofer B, Blettner M, Wahrendorf J. Association between brain tumors and menopausal status. J Natl Cancer Inst 1992;84:1346.
40. Glick RP, Penny D, Hart A. The Pre-Operative and Post-Operative Management of the Brain Tumor Patient. In RA Morantz, JW Walsh (eds), Brain Tumors. New York: Marcel Dekker, 1994;345.
41. The National Radiological Protection Board ad hoc Advisory Group on Nuclear Magnetic Resonance Clinical Imaging. Revised guidelines on acceptable limits of exposure during nuclear magnetic resonance clinical imaging. Br J Radiol 1983;56:974.
42. Collaborative Group on Antenatal Steroid Therapy. Effects of antenatal dexamethasone administration in the infant: long-term follow-up. J Pediatr 1984;104:259.
43. Evans MJ, Chrausas GP, Mann DW, et al. Pharmacologic suppression of the fetal adrenal gland *in utero*. JAMA 1985;253:1015.
44. Bain MD, Copas DK, Landon MJ, et al. *In vivo* permeability of the human placenta to inulin and mannitol. J Physiol 1988;399:313.
45. Basso A, Fernandez A, Althabe O, et al. Passage of mannitol from mother to amniotic fluid and fetus. Obstet Gynecol 1977;49:628.
46. Harris JR, Morrow M, Bonadonna G. Cancer of the Breast. In VT DeVita, S Hellman, SA Rosenberg (eds), Cancer Principles and Practice of Oncology (4th ed). Philadelphia: Lippincott, 1993;1264.
47. Cifuentes N, Pickren JW. Metastases from carcinoma of mammary gland: an autopsy study. J Surg Oncol 1979;11:193.
48. Anderson NE. Neurological Complications of Breast Cancer. In RG Wiley (ed), Neurological Complications of Cancer. New York: Marcel Dekker, 1995;311.
49. Hall SM, Buzdar AU, Blumenschein GR. Cranial nerve palsies in metastatic breast cancer due to osseous metastasis without intracranial involvement. Cancer 1983;52:180.
50. Greenberg H, Deck M, Vikram B. Metastasis to the base of the skull: clinical findings in 43 patients. Neurology 1981;31:530.

51. Tsukada Y, Fouad A, Pickren JW, et al. Central nervous system metastasis from breast carcinoma. Autopsy study. Cancer 1983;52:2349.
52. Boogerd W, Vos VW, Hart AAM, et al. Brain metastases in breast cancer: natural history, prognostic factors, and outcome. J Neurooncol 1993;15:165.
53. Cairncross JG, Kim J-H, Posner JB. Radiation therapy for brain metastases. Ann Neurol 1980;7:529.
54. Distefano A, Yap HY, Hortobagyi GN, et al. The natural history of breast cancer patients with brain metastases. Cancer 1979;44:1913.
55. Dethy S, Piccart MJ, Paesmans M, et al. History of brain and epidural metastases from breast cancer in relation with the disease evolution outside the central nervous system. Eur Neurol 1995;35:38.
56. Batchelor T, DeAngelis LM. Medical management of cerebral metastases. Neurosurg Clin North Am 1996;7:435.
57. Patchell RA, Tibbs PA, Walsh JW, et al. A randomized trial of surgery in the treatment of single metastases to the brain. N Engl J Med 1990;322:494.
58. Mehta MP, Rozental JM, Levin AB, et al. Defining the role of radiosurgery in the management of brain metastases. Int J Radiat Oncol Biol Phys 1992;24:619.
59. Rosner D, Nemoto T, Lane WW. Chemotherapy induces regression of brain metastases in breast carcinoma. Cancer 1986;58:832.
60. Stewart DJ, Dahrouge S. Response of brain metastases from breast cancer to megestrol acetate: a case report. J Neurooncol 1995;24:299.
61. Bach F, Bjerregaard B, Soletormos G, et al. Diagnostic value of cerebrospinal fluid cytology in comparison with tumor marker activity in central nervous system metastases secondary to breast cancer. Cancer 1993;72:2376.
62. Boogerd W, Hart AAM, van der Sande JJ, et al. Meningeal carcinomatosis in breast cancer. Cancer 1991;67:1685.
63. Yap HY, Yap BS, Tashima CK, et al. Meningeal carcinomatosis in breast cancer. Cancer 1978;42:283.
64. Wasserstrom WR, Glass JP, Posner JB. Diagnosis and treatment of leptomeningeal metastases from solid tumors: experience with 90 patients. Cancer 1982;49:759.
65. Glass JP, Melamed M, Chernik NL, et al. Malignant cells in cerebrospinal fluid (CSF): the meaning of a positive CSF cytology. Neurology 1979;29:1369.
66. Grossman SA, Trump DL, Chen DCP, et al. Cerebrospinal fluid flow abnormalities in patients with neoplastic meningitis. Am J Med 1982;73:641.
67. Glantz M, Hall WA, Cole BF, et al. Diagnosis, management, and survival of patients with leptomeningeal cancer based on cerebrospinal fluid flow studies. Cancer 1995;75:2919.
68. Hitchens R, Bell D, Woods R, et al. A prospective randomized trial of single-agent versus combination chemotherapy in meningeal carcinomatosis. J Clin Oncol 1987;5:1655.
69. Hill ME, Richards MA, Gregory WM, et al. Spinal cord compression in breast cancer: a review of 70 cases. Br J Cancer 1993;68:969.
70. Gilbert RW, Kim J-H, Posner JB. Epidural spinal cord compression from metastatic tumor: diagnosis and treatment. Ann Neurol 1979;3:40.

71. Stark RJ, Henson RA, Evans SJW. Spinal metastases. A retrospective survey from a general hospital. Brain 1982;105:189.
72. Posner JB. Neurologic Complications of Cancer. Philadelphia: FA Davis, 1995.
73. Boogerd W, van der Sande JJ, Kroger R. Early diagnosis and treatment of spinal epidural metastasis in breast cancer: a prospective study. J Neurol Neurosurg Psychiatry 1992;55:1188.
74. Marangano E, Latini P, Checcaglini F, et al. Radiation therapy of spinal cord compression caused by breast cancer: report of a prospective trial. Int J Radiat Oncol Biol Phys 1992;24:301.
75. Assa J. The intercostobrachial nerve in radical mastectomy. J Surg Oncol 1974;6:123.
76. Vecht CJ, van de Brand HJ, Wajer OJ. Post-axillary dissection pain in breast cancer due to a lesion of the intercostobrachial nerve. Pain 1989;38:171.
77. Watson CP, Evans RJ, Watt VR. The post mastectomy pain syndrome and the effect of topical capsaicin. Pain 1989;38:177.
78. Graus F, Vega F, Delattre JY, et al. Plasmapharesis and antineoplastic treatment in central nervous system paraneoplastic syndromes with antineuronal autoantibodies. Neurology 1992;42:536.
79. Cher LM, Hochberg FH, Teruya J, et al. Therapy for paraneoplastic neurologic syndromes in six patients with protein A column immunoadsorption. Cancer 1995;75:1678.
80. Escadero D, Barnadas A, Codina M, et al. Anti-Ri-associated paraneoplastic neurologic disorder without opsoclonus in a patient with breast cancer. Neurology 1993;43:1605.
81. Folli F, Solimena M, Cofiell R, et al. Autoantibodies to a 128-kd synaptic protein in three women with the stiff-man syndrome and breast cancer. N Engl J Med 1993;328:546.
82. Corn BW, Greven KM, Randall ME, et al. The efficacy of cranial irradiation in ovarian cancer metastatic to the brain: analysis of 32 cases. Obstet Gynecol 1995;86:955.
83. Rodriguez GC, Soper JT, Berchuck A, et al. Improved palliation of cerebral metastases in epithelial ovarian cancer using a combined modality approach including radiation therapy, chemotherapy, and surgery. J Clin Oncol 1992;10:1553.
84. Geisler JP, Geisler HE. Brain metastases in epithelial ovarian carcinoma. Gynecol Oncol 1995;57:246.
85. Fadul CE. Neurological Complications of Genitourinary Cancer. In RG Wiley (ed), Neurological Complications of Cancer. New York: Marcel Dekker, 1995;373.
86. Khalil AM, Yamout BI, Tabbal SD, et al. Case report and review of literature: leptomeningeal relapse in epithelial ovarian cancer. Gynecol Oncol 1994;54:227.
87. Peterson K, Rosenblum MK, Kotanides H, et al. Paraneoplastic cerebellar degeneration. A clinical analysis of 55 anti-Yo antibody positive patients. Neurology 1992;42:1931.

88. Hudson CN, Curling M, Potsides P, et al. Paraneoplastic syndromes in patients with ovarian neoplasia. J R Soc Med 1993;86:202.
89. Freilich RJ, Balmaceda C, Seidman AD, et al. Motor neuropathy due to docetaxel and paclitaxel. Neurology 1996;47:115.
90. Sahenk Z, Barohn R, New P, et al. Taxol neuropathy. Arch Neurol 1994;51:726.
91. Perry JR, Warner E. Transient encephalopathy after paclitaxel infusion. Neurology 1996;46:1596.
92. Forsyth PAJ, Cascino TL. Neurological Complications of Chemotherapy. In RG Wiley (ed), Neurological Complications of Cancer. New York: Marcel Dekker, 1995;241.
93. Robinson WR, Muderspach LI. Case report. Spinal cord compression in metastatic cervical cancer. Gynecol Oncol 1993;48:269.
94. Athanassiou A, Begent RHJ, Newlands ES, et al. Central nervous system metastases of choriocarcinoma. Cancer 1983;52:1728.
95. Weed JC, Woodward KT, Hammond CB. Choriocarcinoma metastatic to the brain: therapy and prognosis. Semin Oncol 1982;9:208.
96. Seigle JM, Caputy AJ, Manz HJ, et al. Multiple oncotic intracranial aneurysms and cardiac metastasis from choriocarcinoma: case report and review of the literature. Neurosurgery 1987;20:39.

CHAPTER 5

Multiple Sclerosis

Michael C. Irizarry

Multiple sclerosis (MS) is an inflammatory demyelinating disease of the central nervous system (CNS) characterized pathologically by plaques of perivascular lymphocytic infiltration, demyelination, oligodendrocyte death, gliosis, aberrant remyelination, and oligodendrocyte proliferation [1]. Recurrent attacks of neurologic symptoms (including paresthesias, weakness, vision loss [optic neuritis], diplopia, incoordination, gait difficulties, and dysarthria) reflect involvement of different parts of the CNS. During and following attacks, neurologic examination can demonstrate sensory, reflex, motor, cerebellar, oculomotor, optic nerve, gait, or cognitive deficits [2]. Cerebrospinal fluid (CSF) findings in clinically definite MS include elevated protein (in 25%), mild lymphocytic pleocytosis (<20 per µl), increased gamma-globulin (in 60–75%), increased CSF IgG index (in 80–90%), and the presence of oligoclonal bands by immunoglobulin electrophoresis (in up to 90%). Abnormalities in central conduction time can be detected in visual-evoked potentials (in 75% of definite MS), brain stem auditory-evoked potentials (in 67%), and somatosensory-evoked potentials (in 77%) [2]. Magnetic resonance imaging (MRI) is the most sensitive imaging modality for MS, demonstrating multiple T2-hyperintense white matter lesions, particularly in the periventricular regions; lesions may be observed in the brain stem, cerebellum, and spinal cord. Gadolinium enhancement has been correlated with active inflammation [3].

MS occurs more frequently in women, although the specific treatments for attacks and their complications are generally similar for men and women. This chapter reviews issues specific to women with MS, including epidemiology; contraception; menstrual, sexual, and reproductive endocrine function; and pregnancy. Immunomodulatory and symptomatic treatment of MS is briefly reviewed.

Epidemiology

The epidemiology of MS has been extensively studied throughout the world [4–7]. The prevalence appears to increase with increasing geographic longitude in both the northern and southern hemispheres, with rates in the United States of over 50 per 100,000. In Olmsted County, Minnesota, the prevalence rates were 167 per 100,000, with incidence rates of 7–8 per 100,000 per year [7]. Despite different prevalence and incidence rates throughout the world, studies consistently demonstrate that MS onset is rare before puberty, peaks in the third decade, then declines after the fourth decade [6]. Epidemiologic studies also show a predominance of MS in women, with a cumulative female-to-male ratio of 1.76 to 1.00 in a summary of 30 incidence/prevalence studies [8]. This ratio is even higher in early-onset cases (<20 years old) and late-onset cases (>45 years old), suggesting a possible relation to puberty and menopause. The median age of onset may be slightly older in males; in Olmsted County population-based studies, the median age of onset was 34.3 years for males and 32.4 years for females [5].

An early study of MS patients in England by McAlpine found no difference in the attack rate between males and females, with average yearly attack rates of 0.38 in 155 males and 0.40 in 238 females. The gender ratio, with female predominance, was similar in relapsing-remitting and chronic progressive disease; 60.3% of the 146 chronic progressive patients and 60.7% of the 268 relapsing-remitting patients were female [9]. Although many investigators have found no relationship between sex and prognosis, several studies suggest that male sex is an unfavorable prognostic factor for long-term outcome in MS [10], and that males are over-represented in some groups of chronic progressive MS patients [11, 12]. In 197 patients in southwestern Ontario followed from inception of disease, male sex was associated with progressive disease at onset, cerebellar involvement, and adverse outcome [12]. Survival of women with MS was greater than that of men with MS in the Olmsted County study [2].

Idiopathic optic neuritis also has a female predominance. A population-based study in Olmsted County, Minnesota, found gender significantly associated with prevalence (relative risk for women compared to men 2.47, 95% CI 1.65–3.68) and incidence (relative risk 2.07, 95% CI 1.46–2.92). The overall age-adjusted prevalence for women was 163.9 per 100,000, compared to 65.4 per 100,000 for men. The age-adjusted incidence rates from 1985 to 1991 were 7.5 per 100,000 per year for women and 2.6 per 100,000 per year for men. Gender was not an independent risk factor for the subsequent development of MS after idiopathic optic neuritis. The risk of developing MS over 10 years of follow-up by life-table analysis was 40% for women and 38% for men [13].

The risk of transmission of MS from parent to child appears greater for a mother with MS than for a father. Family history data from a Vancouver clinic found that a female child had a 3.71 ± 0.97% risk of developing MS when her mother was affected, compared to a risk of 2.00 ± 0.81% when her father was affected; the corresponding risks for a male child were 3.84 ± 1.42% and 0.79 ± 0.79% [14]. This was relative to a background lifetime prevalence of 0.1–0.2% [15].

The reasons for this female predominance, which is also seen in other immune-mediated diseases such as systemic lupus erythematosus, rheumatoid arthritis, and myasthenia gravis, is unclear and likely reflects the complex interactions between genetic, hormonal, and immunologic factors [16]. Based on experimental models, hormonal influences have been suggested in the susceptibility to and course of MS. Immunization of animals with encephalitogenic emulsion (containing white matter, spinal cord, or myelin basic protein) can induce a monophasic or relapsing-remitting central demyelinating process, known as experimental allergic encephalomyelitis (EAE). EAE has been used as a model of MS. Oral contraceptives (OCPs) [17], pregnancy [18], estrogens [19, 20], and progestins [21] have been able to prevent or decrease the manifestations of EAE in some models. Sex hormones can influence measures of immune system function in animals. Immune function also differs between men and women, with females having a greater immune response with increased T-suppressor cells. Sex variation in the distribution of HLA haplotypes, in particular increased representation of HLA-DR2 in female MS patients, has also been implicated in MS risk [16].

Oral Contraceptives

OCP use does not have adverse effects on the incidence or overall prognosis of MS. In a prospective English study of 17,032 married women between the ages of 25–39 who were enrolled from 1968 to 1974, 63 women developed MS by 1991. The risk of developing MS was not significantly related to OCP use, parity, history of low–birth weight babies, miscarriages, or pregnancy terminations [22]. A study conducted from 1975 to 1977 of 179 MS patients in Southern Lower Saxony, Germany, found that 26% had used OCPs for at least 3 months, and that 21% of the 92 women of reproductive age were using OCPs. There was no significant effect of OCP use on the degree of disability [23]. Thus, women with MS can be maintained on OCPs, although decreased mobility with the consequent risk of thromboembolism may be a relative contraindication [22]. Higher doses of estrogen (50 µg) or supplemental methods of birth control may be required for suppression of ovulation when taking medications such as antibiotics (rifampin, ampicillin, tetracycline, griseofulvin) or anticonvulsants (phenytoin, carbamazepine, phenobarbital) that can decrease the effectiveness of estrogen [24, 25]. The extent of disability in the disease can affect the use of alternative methods of contraception, such as motor impairment limiting use of a diaphragm or impaired vaginal sensation limiting the safety of an intrauterine device [26]. Furthermore, immunosuppression increases the risk of pelvic inflammatory disease associated with the use of an intrauterine device [25].

Reproductive Endocrine Function

There are few studies examining reproductive endocrine function in MS. Irregular menstrual cycles have been reported in 14–15% of MS patients, a figure comparable to that found in the general population [27, 28]. After the onset of MS, three of 34 patients in one study reported development of irregular menstrual cycles, and one patient reported amenorrhea in association with weight loss [29]. Altered hormone secretion within the pituitary-gonadal axis in 14 patients with MS compared to 14 patients with migraine was suggested by endocrine evaluation. Despite normal menstrual patterns and fertility, MS patients had statistically significant increases in mean serum prolactin, follicle-stimulating hormone (FSH), luteinizing hormone (LH), total and free testosterone, 5α-dihydrotestosterone, and Δ⁴-androstenedione, with decreased levels of estrone sulfate. Steroid hormone-binding globulin, estrone, estradiol-17β, dehydroepiandrosterone sulfate, and free estradiol levels were not significantly different [30]. No abnormality in androgen concentrations (testosterone, 5α-dihydrotestosterone, and Δ⁴-androstenedione) was found in another study of 11 MS patients [31]. Basal and stimulatory values of LH and FSH were normal in a study of 16 female patients with MS, although one woman had primary amenorrhea [28].

Immunosuppressive therapy for MS has been associated with precocious menopause: 17 of 38 women who received intensive immunosuppression with cyclophosphamide and prednisone developed amenorrhea with hypergonadotropic hypoestrogenism at an age of 36 ± 1.6 years [29]. It has been suggested that high-dose estrogen OCPs may reduce the risk of immunosuppression-induced amenorrhea [29]. Immunosuppression may also increase the risk of cervical dysplasia and neoplasia [32, 33]; therefore, regular 6–12 month gynecologic examination, breast examination, and Papanicolaou (Pap) smear have been recommended for women on these medications [34].

Severity of symptoms of MS may change with menstruation, menopause, and estrogen replacement therapy. The effect of the menstrual cycle on MS symptoms is variable. Some females with MS may feel worse during menstruation and have exacerbations of their disease at this time. OCP or estrogen (Premarin) treatment has anecdotally improved menstruation-related cyclic exacerbations [35]. A group of 90 premenopausal MS patients recorded daily whether symptoms were unchanged, worse, or improved. A tendency for improvement during menstruation and the first half of the menstrual cycle with deterioration in the second half of the menstrual cycle was reported [9]. A questionnaire-based study reported that nine of 11 premenopausal women experienced worsening in the pre-menstrual phase, seven of 13 postmenopausal women experienced worsening with climacteric, and six of eight postmenopausal women reported improvement with hormone replacement therapy [36]. In conjunction with the reported decreased activity of the disease during pregnancy, these data support a beneficial effect of relative increased estrogen levels in MS.

Sexual Dysfunction

Clinic-based studies suggest that 45–74% of women with MS experience sexual dysfunction. After the diagnosis of MS, 35–60% of women reported decreased libido, and 54–62% reported decreased sexual activity. Specific causes of sexual dysfunction included problems with vaginal lubrication (21–36%), disturbances of orgasm (33–48%), decreased vaginal sensation (28–48%), fatigue (29–68%), and spasticity (12–24%) [37–42]. These clinic-based samples may overestimate the prevalence of sexual dysfunction. A population-based prevalence cohort of 122 women with MS reported a lower prevalence of sexual dysfunction, with 9.9% reporting decreased libido and 10.5% reporting disturbances of orgasm [43]. Sexual dysfunction has been consistently associated with urinary dysfunction [39, 41, 42], suggesting that spinal cord plaques may be responsible. Association with depression [41], bowel dysfunction [39, 40, 42], spasticity [40], fatigue, and weakness of the pelvic floor [38, 42] have been found in some studies. Other studies have not confirmed the association with bowel dysfunction [41], depression [40], or fatigue [40, 41]. No association was found with duration or type of disease, recent exacerbations, or disability score [37, 39, 41]. Sexual dysfunction may improve with corticosteroid treatment of exacerbations [41], or spontaneously after an exacerbation of MS [38]. Clarifying the relationship of the sexual dysfunction with the course and physical manifestations of MS in particular patients can suggest appropriate therapies, which include informal discussions with the patient and spouse, formal counseling, vaginal creams, specific sexual stimulators, specific coital positions, alternative methods of sexual activity, pelvic floor muscle training, and medications (carbamazepine, amitriptyline, and topical anesthetics) for dysesthesias or hyperesthesias [38, 41, 44].

Pregnancy

There is no apparent effect of MS on fertility, course of pregnancy, labor and delivery, spontaneous abortions, stillbirths, fetal malformations, complications of pregnancy and delivery, or mean birth dimensions of the baby

[25, 45]. The risk of developing MS is not associated with parity [22]. Like rheumatoid arthritis, MS has been associated with gestational remissions and postpartum relapses. A meta-analysis of six retrospective studies noted a decreased relapse rate during the gestational period as compared to non-pregnancy years (mean relative risk 0.78 compared to the same patient in nonpregnancy years), without a predilection for attacks to occur during any particular trimester. An increase in relapse rate in the 3 months postpartum compared to nonpregnancy years was also found (mean relative risk 3.9 compared to same patient when not pregnant) [46]. The corresponding relapse rate during pregnancy was 0.14 per year, and for the 3 months postpartum 1.0 per year, significantly different from expected relapse rates of 0.19–0.23 per year [46, 47]. As these were retrospective studies, however, there are problems with patient selection, assessment of relapses and disability, and biases toward patients with more active disease [47].

Recent prospective studies have attempted to address these confounders. A study of 14 pregnancies in 14 relapsing-remitting MS patients from a prospectively followed clinic population found relapse rates of 0.48 per year during pregnancy and 1.1 per year in the 6 months postpartum, with only the latter value being significantly different from the overall relapse rate during the entire 3-year follow-up period (0.48 per year) [45]. A larger clinic-based study of 125 women with relapsing-remitting MS in which 49 pregnancies occurred, confirmed the increased relapse rate in the 3 months postpartum (1.62 ± 0.38 per year) compared to the baseline non-pregnant, non-postpartum period (0.51 ± 0.08 per year); however, the rate during each trimester of pregnancy was not different from baseline, ranging from 0.61 ± 0.27 to 0.84 ± 0.32 per year [48]. Fifty-eight pregnancies in a longitudinally followed clinic population of 47 women with MS found no statistically significant differences in the distribution of relapses among each trimester and the following two 3-month periods postpartum, although the trend was toward decreasing relapse rate over the course of pregnancy. The relapse rate in the first trimester was 0.57 per year, second trimester 0.31, and third trimester 0.16, with an increase in the 3 months postpartum (relapse rate 0.72 per year). The study did not differentiate between the different subtypes of MS evolution [49]. Serial MRIs in two patients with MS before, during, and after pregnancy demonstrated a reduction in active lesions during the second half of pregnancy followed by an increase in the first months postpartum, despite no change in neurologic examination. Active lesions were defined as new lesions or enlargement of pre-existing lesions relative to the prior scan [50]. Pregnancy does not appear to increase the lifetime relapse rate or affect long-term disability [46, 48, 49, 51, 52], nor is the risk of onset of MS increased during pregnancy months [9, 52]. Breast-feeding does not affect the risk of postpartum deterioration [53, 54]. Given the 20–40% risk of a postpartum exacerbation, adequate rest, reduction of stress, assistance with infant care and night feedings, and a 3-month maternity leave from work have been recommended [34].

Treatment of gestational relapses must minimize the risk of fetal injury. Immunosuppression with azathioprine, cyclosporine, and cyclophosphamide should be avoided, and patients on such medications should avoid becoming pregnant. The administration of such medications during the first weeks of pregnancy may be a medical indication for interruption of pregnancy [26]. Mild exacerbations should not be treated, and for severe exacerbations, short-term, high-dose corticosteroids have been recommended; after such treatments, infants should be observed for signs of hypoadrenalism [46]. Women who have been treated for over 2 weeks with steroids in the year before delivery may require steroid coverage, 100 mg of hydrocortisone administered intramuscularly (IM) every 8 hours, during labor and delivery [25]. Interferon beta-1b and interferon beta-1a are contraindicated in pregnant or nursing women, but may be started soon after delivery in non-nursing mothers to decrease the risk of postpartum relapses [55].

Medications should be minimized during pregnancy. Ampicillin and nitrofurantoin may be used to treat urinary tract infection (UTI) during pregnancy or as prophylaxis in the patient with a strong history of UTI requiring catheterization [25]. Breast-feeding is relatively contraindicated in patients taking immunosuppressive drugs because of the risk of bone marrow or adrenal suppression from medications secreted into breast milk [34].

Anesthesia

General anesthesia does not increase the risk of a relapse of MS in the subsequent months. In 88 general anesthetic procedures in 42 patients with MS, one patient had a relapse and one patient had accelerated progression over 1 month postoperatively [56]. Epidural anesthesia also appears as safe as general or local anesthesia during labor, with exacerbations in the 3 months postpartum in five of 14 deliveries with epidural anesthesia, two of five with general anesthesia, and two of 13 with local anesthesia [57]. In another study, only one of 57 MS patients receiving epidural anesthesia experienced a postoperative relapse [58]. Spinal anesthesia was associated with a postoperative exacerbation in one of nine procedures in one series [56] and two of 19 in another [59]; it has generally been avoided because of anecdotal associations with relapses [56].

Treatment

Treatments for MS include immunomodulatory therapy and symptomatic treatment of complications. Traditionally, corticosteroids have been used to ameliorate acute attacks of relapsing-remitting MS, either in the form of IM adrenocorticotropic hormone (ACTH), oral prednisone, or intravenous

(IV) methylprednisolone. Dosing regimens are on the order of 80 U IV ACTH followed by an IM taper over 3–4 weeks; prednisone, 80 mg per day for 1 week followed by a taper over 3 weeks; or IV methylprednisolone, 1 g for 3 days then tapered over a week [60]. IV methylprednisolone has generally been favored over ACTH [61–63] and oral prednisone alone [64], with up to 85% of patients showing significant improvement, some as early as 3–5 days into treatment with methylprednisolone [65, 66]. Despite initial improvement, corticosteroid treatment does not appear to affect the long-term course of the disease [67]. IV methylprednisolone pulses may have some benefit in chronic progressive disease [68].

While there are relatively few side effects with short-term courses of corticosteroids, patients should be followed for the possible unmasking of UTIs, development of oral and vaginal candidiasis, transient glycosuria and hypertension, hypokalemia, gastritis, acne, pedal edema, and mood changes [69]. Before the first treatment, patients should be screened with complete blood count (CBC) with differential, electrolytes, chemistries, purified-protein derivative screen, chest x-ray, blood pressure, fasting blood sugar, and urinalysis. CBC, electrolytes, and glucose may be rechecked 48 hours after treatment is initiated [60]. Long-term tr_atment with oral corticosteroids is of no benefit in chronic progressive MS and is associated with significant steroid toxicity [70, 71]. Steroid-dependent patients are at risk for obesity, hyperlipidemia, osteoporosis, aseptic necrosis of the hip, glucose intolerance, menstrual irregularities, adrenal suppression, edema, hypertension, gastric complications, skin changes, cataracts, glaucoma, and opportunistic infections.

Immunomodulatory therapy with interferon beta-1b, 0.25 mg (8 million IU) subcutaneously every other day, has been demonstrated to reduce the exacerbation rate, severity of relapses, and MRI-measured progression in relapsing-remitting MS [72, 73]. The medication is well tolerated with the most common adverse effects being flulike symptoms, usually manageable with acetaminophen or nonsteroidal anti-inflammatory medications, and local injection-site reactions. It is absolutely contraindicated in pregnant or nursing mothers and in women attempting to become pregnant [55]. Interferon beta-1a, 30 μg, is given as a weekly IM dose. Other immunomodulatory therapy by oral myelin tolerization or treatment with copolymer I is under investigation.

Cytotoxic agents such as cyclophosphamide [74, 75], azathioprine [76–78], and cyclosporine [79, 80] have been used in chronic progressive MS. Chronic azathioprine has been used in doses of 150 mg per day in association with a prednisone taper. A protocol has been developed for a 3-week course of cyclophosphamide, 400–500 mg daily, in association with ACTH [60]; however, booster therapy of 700 mg/m^2 every 2 months may be required to maintain clinical effect [81]. Methotrexate, 7.5 mg per week orally, has been used in secondarily progressive MS [82]. Clinical trials of these cytotoxic agents have demonstrated a modest clinical effect at best, often with a significant incidence of adverse effects. Patients treated with these medications must be extensively monitored for complications from immunosuppression, bone marrow suppression, hepatotoxicity, hemorrhagic cystitis (cyclophosphamide), risk of malignancy, and teratogenesis. The risks of menstrual disturbances and gynecologic malignancies have been reviewed above. These treatments should be administered by physicians familiar with the use of these toxic agents.

Many medications have been used symptomatically in MS including baclofen, diazepam, and dantrolene for spasticity; clonazepam for tremor; carbamazepine for paroxysmal and sensory symptoms; antidepressants for mood and affect disorders; and amantadine for fatigue [83]. Bladder dysfunction is common in both males and females, although symptomatically, females are more likely to have incontinence complaints (urgency and urge incontinence) and males are more likely to have obstructive complaints (hesitancy). Urodynamic patterns of detrusor hyperreflexia, detrusor hypocontractility, or detrusor-sphincter dyssynergia are found in both males and females [84–87]. Urodynamic evaluation can assist in clarifying the mechanism of bladder dysfunction. Medications often used for bladder dysfunction include intranasal desmopressin for nocturia; propantheline, oxybutynin, and imipramine for detrusor hyperreflexia; prazosin and clonidine for dyssynergia; antibiotics for UTI; and urecholine and intermittent catheterization for failure to void [83, 88].

Conclusion

MS disproportionately affects women of reproductive age. The effects of puberty, menstruation, and menopause on the disease are still poorly characterized, as are the effects of the disease on sexual and reproductive endocrine function. Pregnancy does appear to affect exacerbation rate, with fewer exacerbations during pregnancy and increased exacerbations in the three months postpartum. The overall course of the disease is not affected by pregnancy, OCP use, or breast-feeding. MS does not significantly affect pregnancy course or delivery, although physical limitations may affect postnatal care. Medication treatment of MS patients must include close monitoring for risks of immunosuppression, adrenal suppression, bone marrow suppression, neoplasia, and teratogenesis.

References

1. Prineas JW. The Neuropathology of Multiple Sclerosis. In PJ Vinken, GW Bruyn, HL Klawans, et al. (eds), Handbook of Clinical Neurology. Vol. 3, No. 47: Demyelinating Diseases. New York: Elsevier, 1985;213.
2. Swanson JW. Multiple sclerosis: update in diagnosis and review of diagnostic factors. Mayo Clin Proc 1989;64:577.

3. Katz D, Taubenberger JD, Cannella B, et al. Correlation between magnetic resonance imaging findings and lesion development in multiple sclerosis. Ann Neurol 1993;34:661.
4. Kurtzke JF. Epidemiology of Multiple Sclerosis. In PJ Vinken, GW Bruyn, HL Klawans, et al. (eds), Handbook of Clinical Neurology. Vol. 3, No. 47: Demyelinating Diseases. New York: Elsevier, 1985;259.
5. Wynn DR, Rodriguez M, O'Fallon WM, et al. Update on the epidemiology of multiple sclerosis. Mayo Clin Proc 1989;64:808.
6. Martyn CN. The Epidemiology of Multiple Sclerosis. In WB Matthews, A Compston, IV Allen, et al. (eds), McAlpine's Multiple Sclerosis. New York: Churchill Livingstone, 1991;3.
7. Weinshenker BG. Epidemiology of multiple sclerosis. Neurol Clin 1996;14:291.
8. Duquette P, Pleines J, Girard M, et al. The increased susceptibility of women to multiple sclerosis. Can J Neurol Sci 1992;19:466.
9. McAlpine D, Compston N. Some aspects of the natural history of disseminated sclerosis. Q J Med 1952;21:135.
10. Weinshenker BG, Ebers GC. The natural history of multiple sclerosis. Can J Neurol Sci 1987;14:255.
11. Van Lambalgen R, Sanders EACM, D'Amaro J. Sex distribution, age of onset and HLA profiles in two types of multiple sclerosis. A role for sex hormones and microbial infections in the development of autoimmunity? J Neurol Sci 1986;76:13.
12. Weinshenker BG, Rice GPA, Noseworthy JH, et al. The natural history of multiple sclerosis: a geographically based study. 3. Multivariate analysis of predictive factors and models of outcome. Brain 1991;114:1045.
13. Rodriguez M, Siva A, Cross SA, et al. Optic neuritis: a population-based study in Olmsted County, Minnesota. Neurology 1995;45:244.
14. Sadovnick AD, Baird PA, Ward RH. Multiple sclerosis: updated risks for relatives. Am J Med Genet 1988;29:533.
15. Sadovnick AD. Familial recurrence risks and inheritance of multiple sclerosis. Curr Opin Neurol Neurosurg 1993;6:189.
16. Duquette P, Girard M. Hormonal factors in susceptibility to multiple sclerosis. Curr Opin Neurol Neurosurg 1993;6:195.
17. Arnason BG, Richman DP. Effect of oral contraceptives on experimental demyelinating disease. Arch Neurol 1969;21:103.
18. Evron S, Brenner T, Abramsky O. Suppressive effect of pregnancy on the development of experimental allergic encephalomyelitis in rabbits. Am J Reprod Immunol 1984;5:109.
19. Jansson L, Olsson T, Holmdahl R. Estrogen induces a potent suppression of experimental autoimmune encephalomyelitis and collagen-induced arthritis in mice. J Neuroimmunol 1994;53:203.
20. Trooster WJ, Teelken AW, Kampinga J, et al. Suppression of acute experimental allergic encephalomyelitis by the synthetic sex hormone 17-alpha-ethinylestradiol: an immunological study in the Lewis rat. Int Arch Allergy Immunol 1993;102:133.

21. Greig ME, Gibbons AJ, Elliott GA. A comparison of the effects of melengestrol acetate and hydrocortisone acetate on experimental allergic encephalomyelitis in rats. J Pharmacol Exp Ther 1970;173:85.

22. Villard-Mackintosh L, Vessey MP. Oral contraceptives and reproductive factors in multiple sclerosis incidence. Contraception 1993;47:161.

23. Poser S, Raun NE, Wikstrom J, et al. Pregnancy, oral contraceptives, and multiple sclerosis. Acta Neurologica Scand 1979;59:108.

24. Stockley I. Interactions with oral contraceptives. Pharm J 1976;216:140.

25. Birk K, Rudick R. Pregnancy and multiple sclerosis. Arch Neurol 1986;43:719.

26. Poser S. Management of Patients with Multiple Sclerosis. In PJ Vinken, GW Bruyn, HL Klawans, et al. (eds), Handbook of Clinical Neurology. Vol. 3, No. 47: Demyelinating Diseases. New York: Elsevier, 1985;147.

27. Poser S, Kreikenbaum K, König A, et al. Endokrinologische Befunde bei Patientinnen mit multipler Sklerose. Geburtshilfe Frauenheilkd 1981;41:353.

28. Klapps P, Seyfert S, Fischer T, et al. Endocrine function in multiple sclerosis. Acta Neurol Scand, 1992;85:353.

29. Linssen WHJP, Notermans NC, Hommes OR, et al. Amenorrhea after immunosuppressive treatment of multiple sclerosis. Acta Neurol Scand 1987;76:204.

30. Grinsted L, Heltberg A, Hagen C, et al. Serum sex hormone and gonadotropin concentrations in premenopausal women with multiple sclerosis. J Intern Med 1989;226:241.

31. Dougados M, Nahoul K, Benhamou L, et al. Étude des androgenes plasmatiques chez les femme atteintes de maladies auto-immunes. Rev Rhum 1984;51:145.

32. Sillman F, Stanek A, Sedlis A, et al. The relationship between human papillomavirus and lower genital intraepithelial neoplasia in immunosuppressed women. Am J Obstet Gynecol 1984;150:300.

33. Schneider V, Kay S, Lee HM. Immunosuppression as a high-risk factor in the development of condyloma acuminatum and squamous neoplasia of the cervix. Acta Cytol 1983;27:220.

34. Rudick RA, Birk KA. Multiple Sclerosis and Pregnancy. In PJ Goldstein, BJ Stern (eds), Neurologic Disorders of Pregnancy. Mount Kisco, NY: Futura, 1992;165.

35. McFarland HR. The management of multiple sclerosis. 3. Apparent suppression of symptoms by an estrogen-progestin compound. Mo Med 1969;66:209.

36. Smith R, Studd JWW. A pilot study of the effect upon multiple sclerosis of the menopause, hormone replacement therapy and the menstrual cycle. J R Soc Med 1992;85:612.

37. Lilius HG, Valtonen EJ, Wikstrom J. Sexual problems in patients suffering from multiple sclerosis. J Chron Dis 1976;29:643.

38. Lundberg PO. Sexual dysfunction in female patients with multiple sclerosis. Int Rehab Med 1981;3:32.

39. Minderhoud JM, Leemhuis JG, Kremer J, et al. Sexual disturbances arising from multiple sclerosis. Acta Neurol Scand 1984;70:299.

40. Valleroy ML, Kraft GH. Sexual dysfunction in multiple sclerosis. Arch Phys Med Rehabil 1984;65:125.
41. Mattson D, Petrie M, Srivastava DK, et al. Multiple sclerosis: sexual dysfunction and its response to medications. Arch Neurol 1995;52:862.
42. Hulter BM, Lundberg PO. Sexual function in women with advanced multiple sclerosis. J Neurol Neurosurg Psychiatry 1995;59:83.
43. Rodriguez M, Siva A, Ward J, et al. Impairment, disability, and handicap in multiple sclerosis: a population-based study in Olmsted County, Minnesota. Neurology 1994;44:28.
44. Szasz G, Paty D, Maurice WL. Sexual dysfunction in multiple sclerosis. Ann N Y Acad Sci 1984;436:443.
45. Worthington J, Jones R, Crawford M, et al. Pregnancy and multiple sclerosis—a 3-year prospective study. J Neurol 1993;241:228.
46. Cook SD, Troiano R, Bansil S, et al. Multiple Sclerosis and Pregnancy. In O Devinsky, E Feldmann, B Hainline (eds), Neurologic Complications of Pregnancy. New York: Raven, 1994;83.
47. Hutchinson M. Pregnancy in multiple sclerosis. J Neurol Neurosurg Psychiatry 1993;56:1043.
48. Roullet E, Verdier-Taillefer M-H, Amarenco P, et al. Pregnancy and multiple sclerosis: a longitudinal study of 125 remittent patients. J Neurol Neurosurg Psychiatry 1993;56:1062.
49. Sadovnick AD, Eisen K, Hashimoto SA, et al. Pregnancy and multiple sclerosis. A prospective study. Arch Neurol 1994;51:1120.
50. van Walderveen MAA, Tas MW, Barkhof F, et al. Magnetic resonance evaluation of disease activity during pregnancy in multiple sclerosis. Neurology 1994;44:327.
51. Poser S, Poser W. Multiple sclerosis and gestation. Neurology 1983;33:1422.
52. Thompson DS, Nelson LM, Burns A, et al. The effects of pregnancy in multiple sclerosis: a retrospective study. Neurology 1986;36:1097.
53. Poser CM, Poser S, Poser W. MS and postpartum stress. Neurology 1984;34:704.
54. Nelson LM, Franklin GM, Jones MC, et al. Risk of multiple sclerosis exacerbation during pregnancy and breast-feeding. JAMA 1988;259:3441.
55. Lublin FD, Whitaker JN, Eidelman BH, et al. Management of patients receiving interferon beta-1b for multiple sclerosis: report of a consensus conference. Neurology 1996;46:12.
56. Bamford C, Sibley W, Laguna J. Anesthesia in multiple sclerosis. Can J Neurol Sci 1978;5:41.
57. Bader AM, Hunt CO, Datta S, et al. Anesthesia for the obstetric patient with multiple sclerosis. J Clin Anesth 1988;1:21.
58. Crawford JS. Epidural anesthesia for patients with chronic neurologic disease. Anesth Analg 1983;62:617.
59. Stenuit J, Marchand P. Les sequelles de rachia anesthisie. Acta Neurol Belg 1968;68:626.
60. Lopez-Bresnahan MV, Hauser SL. Multiple Sclerosis. In RE Rakel (ed), Conn's Current Therapy. Philadelphia: Saunders, 1992;859.

61. Abruzzesse G, Gandolofo C, Loeb C. Bolus methylprednisolone versus ACTH in the treatment of multiple sclerosis. Ital J Neurol Sci 1983;2:169.
62. Barnes MP, Bateman DE, Cleland PG, et al. Intravenous methylprednisolone for multiple sclerosis in relapse. J Neurol Neurosurg Psychiatry 1985;48:157.
63. Thompson AJ, Kennard C, Swash M, et al. Relative efficacy of intravenous methylprednisolone and ACTH in the treatment of acute relapse in MS. Neurology 1989;39:969.
64. Ohno R, Hamaguchi K, Sowa K, et al. High-dose intravenous corticosteroids in the treatment of multiple sclerosis. Jpn J Med 1987;26:212.
65. Durelli L, Cocito D, Riccio A, et al. High-dose intravenous methylprednisolone in the treatment of multiple sclerosis: clinical-immunologic correlations. Neurology 1986;35:238.
66. Milligan NM, Newcome R, Compston DA. A double-blind controlled trial of high dose methylprednisolone in patients with multiple sclerosis. J Neurol Neurosurg Psychiatry 1987;50:511.
67. Compston A. Methylprednisolone and multiple sclerosis. Arch Neurol 1988;45:669.
68. Cazzato G, Mesiano T, Antonello R, et al. Double-blind, placebo-controlled, randomized, crossover trial of high-dose methylprednisolone in patients with chronic progressive form of multiple sclerosis. Eur Neurol 1995;35:93.
69. Lyons PR, Newman PK, Saunders M. Methylprednisolone therapy in multiple sclerosis: a profile of adverse effects. J Neurol Neurosurg Psychiatry 1988;51:285.
70. Miller JHD, Vas CJ, Noronha MJ, et al. Long-term treatment of multiple sclerosis with corticotrophin. Lancet 1967;2:429.
71. Fog T. The long-term treatment of multiple sclerosis with corticoids. Acta Neurol Scand 1965;13:473.
72. IFNB Multiple Sclerosis Study Group. Interferon beta-1b is effective in relapsing-remitting multiple sclerosis: I. Clinical results of a multicenter, randomized, double-blind, placebo-controlled trial. Neurology 1993;43:655.
73. Paty DW, Li DKB. Interferon beta-1b is effective in relapsing-remitting multiple sclerosis: II. MRI analysis results of a multicenter, randomized, double-blind, placebo-controlled trial. Neurology 1993;43:662.
74. Canadian Cooperative Multiple Sclerosis Study Group. The Canadian cooperative trial of cyclophosphamide and plasma exchange in progressive multiple sclerosis. Lancet 1991;337:441.
75. Likosky WH, Fireman B, Elmore R, et al. Intense immunosuppression in chronic progressive multiple sclerosis: the Kaiser Study. J Neurol Neurosurg Psychiatry 1991;54:1055.
76. British and Dutch Multiple Sclerosis Azathioprine Trial Group. Double-masked trial of azathioprine in multiple sclerosis. Lancet 1988;2:179.
77. Ellison GW, Myers LW, Mickey MR, et al. A placebo-controlled, randomized, double-masked, variable dosage, clinical trial of azathioprine with and without methylprednisolone in multiple sclerosis. Neurology 1989;39:1018.
78. Yudkin PL, Ellison GW, Ghezzi A, et al. Overview of azathioprine treatment in multiple sclerosis. Lancet 1991;338:1051.

79. Multiple Sclerosis Study Group. Efficacy and toxicity of cyclosporin in chronic progressive multiple sclerosis: a randomized, double-blinded, placebo-controlled clinical trial. Ann Neurol 1990;27:591.
80. Rudge P, Koetsier JC, Mertin J, et al. Randomised double-blind controlled trial of cyclosporin in multiple sclerosis. J Neurol Neurosurg Psychiatry 1989;52:559.
81. Weiner HL, Mackin GA, Orav EJ, et al. Intermittent cyclophosphamide pulse therapy in progressive multiple sclerosis: final report of the Northeast Cooperative Multiple Sclerosis Treatment Group. Neurology 1993;43:910.
82. Goodkin DE, Rudick RA, Medendorp SV, et al. Low-dose (7.5 mg) oral methotrexate reduces the rate of progression in chronic progressive multiple sclerosis. Ann Neurol 1995;37:30.
83. van Oosten BW, Truyen L, Barkhof F, et al. Multiple sclerosis therapy: a practical guide. Drugs 1995;49:200.
84. Bradley WE, Logothetis JL, Timm GW. Cystometric and sphincter abnormalities in multiple sclerosis. Neurology 1973;23:1131.
85. Andersen JT. Abnormalities of detrusor and sphincter function in multiple sclerosis. Brit J Urol 1976;48:193.
86. Mayo ME, Chetner MP. Lower urinary tract dysfunction in multiple sclerosis. Urology 1992;39:67.
87. Koldewijn EL, Hommes OR, Lemmens WAJG, et al. Relationship between lower urinary tract abnormalities and disease-related parameters in multiple sclerosis. J Urol 1995;154:169.
88. Schapiro RT. Symptom management in multiple sclerosis. Ann Neurol 1994;36(Suppl):S123.

CHAPTER 6

Neuromuscular Disorders

Mark W. Faragher

This chapter provides an overview of the specific features of neuropathies, neuromuscular junction disorders, and muscle disorders in women. The neuromuscular complications of pregnancy are addressed within each section. The chapter concludes with a discussion of the neuromuscular complications of female malignancies.

Generalized Neuropathies

Guillain-Barré Syndrome

The incidence of Guillain-Barré syndrome in the general population is 1.7 cases per 100,000 per year. Incidence is higher in females (2.3 cases per 100,000 per year) than in males (1.2 cases per 100,000 per year). Incidence is higher in older people (3.2 cases per 100,000 per year in the population over age 60) compared to younger people (0.8 cases per 100,000 per year in those under age 18) [1].

Guillain-Barré syndrome may occur in pregnancy [2]. Its incidence during pregnancy is similar to the incidence in women of the same age [3]; however, pregnant women are more prone to respiratory complications from respiratory compromise due to the gravid uterus. Approximately 33% of gravid patients with Guillain-Barré syndrome require mechanical ventilation, compared with 16% of nonpregnant patients. Evidence suggests that mortality and morbidity rates are higher in gravid patients with Guillain-Barré syndrome [3, 4].

The efficacy of plasmapheresis in Guillain-Barré syndrome has been demonstrated in randomized trials [5, 6]. It is a safe treatment in pregnancy [3]. An alternative is the administration of intravenous (IV) gamma globulin.

Chronic Inflammatory Demyelinating Polyneuropathy

Chronic inflammatory demyelinating polyneuropathy (CIDP) may occur de novo in pregnancy [7, 8]. In addition, a patient with pre-existing CIDP is more likely to relapse during pregnancy [9]. When occurring de novo, the onset tends to be in the second half of pregnancy or in the early puerperium [7]. A case of CIDP associated with the use of oral contraceptives (OCPs) has also been reported [10]. The standard therapies of corticosteroids, plasmapheresis, and IV gamma globulin can all be used in pregnancy.

Toxic Neuropathies

An outbreak of acute polyneuropathy affected over 20 young Tamil females in Sri Lanka during 1977–78 [11]. The illness was restricted to girls attaining menarche and women in the postpartum period. The cause of the neuropathy was traced to tricresyl phosphate, which was found to be a contaminant of gingili oil. The illness was limited to these two groups due to local customs. On attaining menarche, the Tamil girls were confined at home and fed a combination of raw eggs and gingili oil. Other Tamils were not exposed to the gingili oil because it was only given in these circumstances due to its high cost. Three women who presented with the illness postpartum had been consuming gingili oil as a tonic according to local Muslim custom.

The Porphyrias

The porphyrias are disorders characterized by the excessive production of porphyrins and porphyrin precursors resulting from specific enzymatic defects in the heme biosynthetic pathway [12]. Neurologic manifestations include sensorimotor and autonomic neuropathies. Synthetic estrogens and progestins may precipitate porphyric crises. In a proportion of women with acute intermittent porphyria, mild to disabling attacks occur in relation to the menstrual cycle, usually in the luteal phase or, less commonly, at ovulation [13]. In some of these patients, long-term suppression of ovarian cyclicity with OCPs has paradoxically produced prolonged remissions. Danazol, a synthetic steroid with weak androgenic activity, is an alternative [14].

Paradoxically, OCP use may produce exacerbations of porphyria in some women [15]. Luteinizing hormone–releasing hormone analogues may provide a rational approach to the therapy of cyclical attacks of acute intermittent porphyria in the future [16].

Cranial Neuropathies

Bell's Palsy

In a series of 446 patients, Bell's palsy was more severe in women than in men [17]. More females than males experienced complete paralysis, contracture, and synkinesis. However, there was no difference in recovery rates between men and women. The calculated incidence of Bell's palsy is 45 cases per 100,000 term pregnancies; for nonpregnant women of the same age group, the calculated incidence is 17 per 100,000 per year [18]. No causative relationship has been demonstrated between toxemia, hypertension, or primigravidity and Bell's palsy. The incidence for the third trimester and early puerperium is 118 per 100,000 per year, which demonstrates that the increased incidence of cases in pregnant women occurs mostly at this time. Gestational diabetes does not account for the excess. Over 60% of the cases in nonpregnant women occur in the first 14 days of the menstrual cycle with peaks on the first and seventh days and near ovulation.

The prognosis for recovery during pregnancy is similar to nongestational Bell's palsy. A 10-day tapering course of prednisone may be safe in the second and third trimesters but is probably best avoided in the first trimester [18]. Protection of the eye and the use of artificial tears and lubricant are important if paresis of the orbicularis oculi is so severe as to leave the cornea exposed.

There have even been reports of lower motor neuron facial palsy occurring in successive pregnancies. Gbolade reported lower motor neuron facial palsy in four consecutive pregnancies in one patient [19].

Upper Extremity Neuropathies

Median Neuropathy at the Wrist

Epidemiology

Carpal tunnel syndrome (CTS) is most common in middle-aged women. In one series the ratio of women to men was approximately 3 to 1 [20]. Phalen stated that most of the women treated were at or near menopause, suggesting that hormonal factors may play a causative role.

Diagnosis

The classic clinical symptoms are numbness or tingling in the median nerve sensory distribution of the hand. Initially this may wake the patient from sleep. The symptoms may be worse while performing certain tasks such as driving or holding a telephone. If the condition progresses, pain may become a symptom in the same median nerve sensory distribution, and weakness and atrophy of the thenar eminence may be noted. Although usually bilateral, the symptoms are often worse in the patient's dominant hand.

Nerve conduction studies (NCS) and electromyography (EMG) are useful in confirming the clinical diagnosis. The criteria for a median nerve lesion at the wrist are well defined [21]. NCS and EMG are particularly useful in atypical patients who may present with pain that radiates proximally.

Pathophysiology

The flexor retinaculum forms the roof of the carpal tunnel. It attaches to the pisiform bone and the hook of the hamate on the medial side, and to the tubercle of the scaphoid and the tubercle of the trapezium on the other. The median nerve travels through the carpal tunnel accompanied by the nine long flexor tendons of the hand. The ulnar nerve and vessels, the palmar cutaneous branches of the median and ulnar nerves, and the tendon of the palmaris longus lie superficial to the flexor retinaculum. The floor of the carpal tunnel is formed by the carpal bones (Figure 6.1).

The median nerve and flexor tendons and their synovial sheaths are tightly packed in the carpal tunnel. Any swelling leads to compromise of the median nerve. Tenosynovitis of the flexor tendons' synovial sheaths is the cause of most cases of idiopathic CTS. Secondary causes include diabetes, hypothyroidism, rheumatoid arthritis, acromegaly, and amyloidosis.

An increase in the wrist depth-to-width ratio, known as the *wrist ratio*, has been correlated with CTS [22]. The wrist ratio is more likely to be abnormal in women than men and may provide a clue as to why women are more often affected by CTS than men.

The cross-section area of the carpal tunnel has been studied using computed tomography (CT) [23]. The proximal carpal tunnel cross-section area (pisiform bone to the tubercle of the scaphoid) of female patients with CTS is significantly smaller than that of female controls, and the cross-section area of female controls is significantly smaller than in male controls. This suggests an association between a small carpal tunnel and symptoms of CTS. The smaller carpal canal cross-section area in females compared with males may explain the female propensity for the condition.

CTS is very common in pregnancy [24]. The typical time of onset is in the third trimester [25]. The cases in Wand's study were all associated with peripheral edema. The condition will usually improve after delivery, so it may be managed conservatively with wrist splints or local steroid injection. Very rarely, carpal tunnel release is required. It has been suggested that pregnant women with CTS and the following additional characteristics are more likely to require surgery: symptoms of CTS before pregnancy, development of symptoms during the first two trimesters, and both a positive Phalen test within less than 30 seconds and a two-point discrimination threshold of more than 6 mm at the tip of the finger [26].

CTS that develops in the puerperium, without previous symptoms during pregnancy, tends to affect older women more than does CTS that develops during pregnancy. One study found that it primarily affected older primiparous women (mean age 31.5) who were breast-feeding, with onset 3 weeks after delivery [27]. It resolves 2–3 weeks after weaning and rarely requires surgery. CTS in the puerperium is not associated with peripheral edema.

CTS has been reported in association with OCP use, providing additional evidence of a hormonal role in the pathogenesis of the condition [28]. OCP use has not been prominently associated with CTS in the 1990s. This is possibly because the original reports described the association in the context of older forms of OCPs, which contained relatively high-dose estrogen and are no longer used.

Treatment

Treatment may be conservative in approach or involve surgery. Conservative treatment involves use of analgesics, anti-inflammatory agents, wrist splints, or steroid injections. Diuretics may be useful when the symptoms are perimenstrual. Surgical treatment is usually used only after conservative treatment has failed or if the CTS is severe. Either open procedures or laparoscopic procedures are performed. Surgery is generally very successful. Acute CTS (for example, in a case of Colles' fracture, which commonly occurs in postmenopausal women) often needs immediate decompression.

Neuralgic Amyotrophy

The term *neuralgic amyotrophy* was coined in 1948 to describe a syndrome of localized neuritis of the shoulder girdle. The essential clinical features are severe shoulder pain followed within hours or days either by weakness in muscles supplied by a single nerve such as the axillary, long thoracic, or anterior interosseous nerve, or upper extremity weakness in the distribution of peripheral nerves or nerve roots. There is generally little sensory involvement [29]. A relationship between pregnancy and neuralgic amyotrophy has been recognized in the rare familial variant. In such families, susceptibility to the condition is inherited in a fashion suggesting an autosomal dominant gene with a high degree of penetrance. Affected individuals have recurrent episodes of focal pain followed by arm weakness, which may be in the distribution of multiple nerve roots, parts of the brachial plexus, or multiple peripheral nerves. In some of these families, affected women are prone to attacks during pregnancy or shortly after delivery [30]. It has also been reported that menarche may increase the frequency of attacks of familial brachial plexopathy [31].

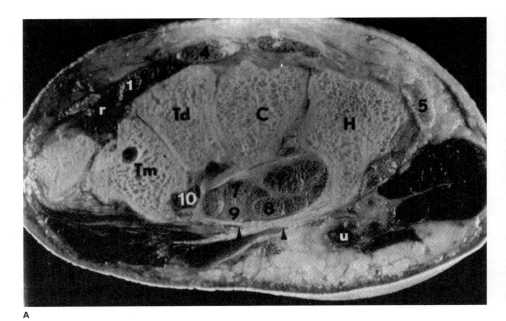

A

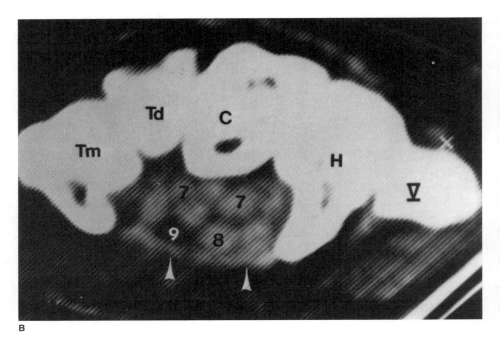

B

FIGURE 6.1. Cross-section illustrations through the carpal tunnel. Transverse sections of the soft tissues and bony structure of the wrist at the level of the hook of the hamate are demonstrated in cadaveric section (A) and with computed tomography (B). (arrowheads = transverse carpal ligament; V = fifth metacarpal; 1 = extensor carpi

Extensor digitorum & indicis tt

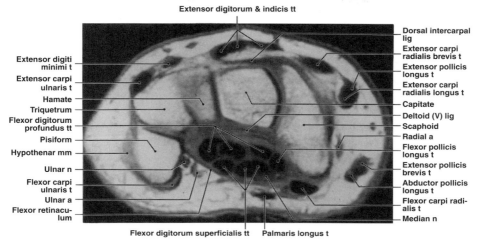

Extensor digiti minimi t
Extensor carpi ulnaris t
Hamate
Triquetrum
Flexor digitorum profundus tt
Pisiform
Hypothenar mm
Ulnar n
Flexor carpi ulnaris t
Ulnar a
Flexor retinaculum

Dorsal intercarpal lig
Extensor carpi radialis brevis t
Extensor pollicis longus t
Extensor carpi radialis longus t
Capitate
Deltoid (V) lig
Scaphoid
Radial a
Flexor pollicis longus t
Extensor pollicis brevis t
Abductor pollicis longus t
Flexor carpi radialis t
Median n

Flexor digitorum superficialis tt   Palmaris longus t

C

Extensor digitorum & indicis tt

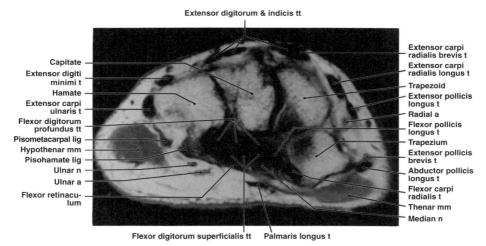

Capitate
Extensor digiti minimi t
Hamate
Extensor carpi ulnaris t
Flexor digitorum profundus tt
Pisometacarpal lig
Hypothenar mm
Pisohamate lig
Ulnar n
Ulnar a
Flexor retinaculum

Extensor carpi radialis brevis t
Extensor carpi radialis longus t
Trapezoid
Extensor pollicis longus t
Radial a
Flexor pollicis longus t
Trapezium
Extensor pollicis brevis t
Abductor pollicis longus t
Flexor carpi radialis t
Thenar mm
Median n

Flexor digitorum superficialis tt   Palmaris longus t

D

radialis longus and brevis; 4 = digital extensors; 5 = extensor carpi ulnaris; 7 = flexor digitorum profundus; 8 = flexor digitorum superficialis; 9 = median nerve; 10 = flexor carpi radialis; C = capitate; H = hamate; Td = trapezoid; Tm = trapezium; r = radial artery; u = ulnar artery.) (Reproduced with permission from RO Cone, R Szabo, D Resnick, et al. Computed tomography of the normal soft tissue of the wrist. Invest Radiol 1983;18:546.) Transverse T1-weighted magnetic resonance images through the carpal tunnel at the level of the pisiform (C) and, more distal to this, at the level of the hamate (D). (a = artery; lig = ligament; mm = muscles; n = nerve; t = tendon; tt = tendons.) (Reproduced with permission from HS Kang, D Resnick. MRI of the Extremities: An Anatomic Atlas. Philadelphia: Saunders, 1991;137.)

In addition to the well-recognized familial form, neuralgic amyotrophy may occur in a sporadic fashion in women during pregnancy [32] and in the postpartum period [33]. One case of sporadic bilateral brachial plexopathy has been described during pregnancy. The patient was a 32-year-old woman who, in the second trimester, developed involvement in the right upper extremity that resolved and then relapsed at 34 weeks, followed by the development of left upper extremity involvement 1 week later. The outcome was poor and associated with psychosocial consequences. In a series of eight women with sporadic postpartum neuralgic amyotrophy, only one had clinical features suggestive of an inherited condition [33].

The course is similar in the spontaneous, familial, and gestational forms. Pain is typically the first symptom and resolves spontaneously within a few weeks. EMG and NCS often show evidence of axonal interruption and motor recovery may take months. No specific therapy is of proven value, although prednisone may help alleviate pain.

In any upper extremity lesion occurring immediately after cesarean section, the differential diagnosis of compression or stretch injury to the brachial plexus during anesthesia must be considered. Another potential cause is intermittent brachial plexopathy secondary to breast engorgement [34].

Contraceptive-Related Neuropathies

Levonorgestrel (Norplant) is an implantable subdermal contraceptive agent that has been available in the United States since 1991. Musculocutaneous nerve lesions have been reported with levonorgestrel subdermal implantation [35]. The symptoms resolved with removal of the subdermal system.

Lower Extremity Neuropathies

Nerve injury in the lower extremity may occur at the level of the spinal root, lumbosacral plexus, or peripheral nerve.

Nonspecific back pain is very common in pregnancy. However, actual nerve root compression from prolapsed disc fragments is rare [36]. Pregnancy may predispose a woman to lumbar disc herniation later in life [37]. Kelsey et al. found that the more live births a woman has, the more likely she is to have subsequent lumbar disc herniation. They suggested the action of the hormone relaxin in the third trimester and mechanical stress as possible causes of this relationship [37].

The lumbosacral plexus may be injured during delivery. Some authors estimate the incidence to be between one in 2,100 and one in 6,400 deliveries [38]. The lesion usually affects the lower portion of the lumbosacral plexus, producing distal weakness with predominant peroneal territory involvement. The nerve lesion probably results from direct pressure by the descending fetal head compressing the lumbosacral trunk and the S1 root

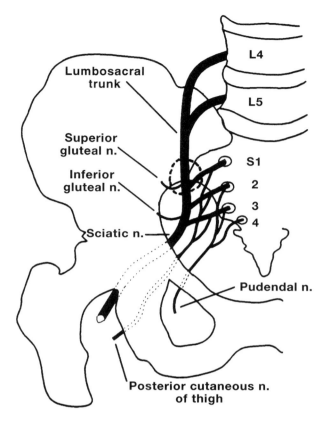

FIGURE 6.2. Diagram of the lumbosacral plexus showing the presumed site of the compressive nerve lesion *(dashed-line circle)*. (Reproduced with permission from TE Feasby, SR Burton, AF Hahn. Obstetrical lumbosacral plexus injury. Muscle Nerve 1992;15:937.)

as it joins the trunk against the rim of the pelvis during the second stage of labor (Figure 6.2). Recovery is variable and depends on the severity of the initial deficit.

Pregnancy is associated with femoral neuropathy [39], iliohypogastric nerve entrapment [40], obturator neuropathy, and lesions of the lateral cutaneous nerve of the thigh; the latter are also known as *meralgia paresthetica* [41]. Femoral neuropathy may occur as a complication of the lithotomy position rather than pregnancy per se.

Childbirth is associated with an array of lower extremity neuropathies. These include injury to the common peroneal nerve from prolonged hyperflexion of the knee due to squatting during natural childbirth [42, 43].

Epidural anesthesia, which is commonly used in obstetric practice, is associated with a small risk (approximately 0.1%) of injury to the spinal cord or nerve roots [44]. Neurologic deficits may be caused by epidural hematomas, particularly in anticoagulated patients; chemical radiculitis or arachnoiditis; direct needle injury to the nerve root; or spinal cord infarc-

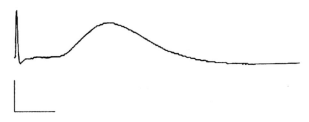

FIGURE 6.3.   A compound muscle-action potential recorded from the external anal sphincter using the St. Mark's electrode to stimulate the pudendal nerve. The horizontal bar represents 2 milliseconds and the vertical bar represents 1,000 mV. For the waveform illustrated, the distal motor latency is 2.1 milliseconds and the amplitude is 1,030 mV.

tion secondary to hypotension. The single nerve root most commonly affected is L2. More extensive lumbosacral polyradiculopathies have been reported. Neurologic complications may be more severe in the presence of spinal stenosis or after inadvertent subarachnoid injection of anesthetic or analgesic agent [45].

Pudendal Nerve

A degree of stress urinary incontinence develops after childbirth in many women. Such urinary incontinence may develop many years after childbirth. Some of these women have fecal incontinence as well. Occult pudendal nerve damage during vaginal delivery has been implicated as an important factor in the pathogenesis of such urinary incontinence [46]. The pudendal nerve forms from the S2, S3, and S4 nerve roots. It innervates perineal skin, levator ani, and the external anal and urinary sphincters. Bilateral pudendal nerve blockade in healthy women reduces the urethral pressure significantly [47]. This observation supports the hypothesis that the pudendal nerve is important in maintaining urinary continence.

The pudendal terminal motor latency is measured from the time of stimulation to the onset of the motor response (Figure 6.3). The technique was first described in 1984 [48]. It is commonly performed with the St. Mark's electrode. A bipolar-stimulating electrode mounted on the tip of the index finger is placed against the ischial spine via the rectum. The recording electrodes are at the base of the palmar side of the index finger and lie against the anal sphincter.

Pudendal nerve terminal motor latency has been studied prospectively in 128 pregnant women [49]. Vaginal delivery resulted in a significant prolongation in the pudendal latency bilaterally in the primiparous women. The pudendal nerve latency did not change in those women treated with elective cesarean section. A heavy fetus and a long second stage of labor correlated with a prolongation in the pudendal latency. Prolonged pudendal nerve motor latency has been shown to be a predictor of fecal incontinence after childbirth [50].

Catamenial Sciatica

Ectopic endometrial tissue (endometriosis) infrequently affects the peripheral nervous system. In this location, as elsewhere, this tissue behaves like normal endometrium, responding to hormonal stimuli and undergoing epithelial sloughing and hemorrhage at the time of menses [12].

Catamenial sciatica is a rare presenting symptom associated with endometriosis. Misdiagnosis can lead to unnecessary surgery such as laminectomy. Initially, the sciatica is perimenstrual, starting 1–2 days before the first day of menstruation and continuing until several days after menses. The pain may involve the buttock and posterior thigh. With progression of the disease, the pain-free period of each cycle may shorten until the pain becomes continuous with exacerbations during menstruation. At this stage there may be leg weakness and even foot drop. The pain is due to perimenstrual hemorrhage into deposits of endometrial tissue deposited along the course of the sciatic nerve [51]. Pelvic CT examination is often distinctive, showing a solid mass at the level of the greater sciatic notch that may enhance with contrast [52]. Magnetic resonance imaging (MRI) may show the lesion as well [53]. Laparoscopy and biopsy enables histologic diagnosis showing characteristic glandular elements. In some cases when endometriosis is not immediately obvious on laparoscopy, the only indication may be the "pocket" sign, in which a pocket of peritoneum is drawn down toward the greater sciatic notch [54].

Medical management with danazol [52] or leuprolide, a gonadotropin releasing–hormone antagonist, is an option [55]. However, surgical exploration of the sciatic nerve in combination with laparoscopy is usually required. Involution of endometriosis may occur in pregnancy. A more radical option offering permanent cure of endometriosis is surgical castration.

Ectopic endometrial tissue may destroy lumbar vertebrae, producing lower back pain, and invade the lumbosacral plexus in the retroperitoneal space [56]. Endometrial tissue located within the spinal canal may produce a combination of central and peripheral nervous system pathologies. In one case, a 26-year-old woman suffered cyclic L1–2 pain and subarachnoid hemorrhage of unknown etiology. Eventually a myelogram showed a mass at the level of L1–2 that, on laminectomy, proved to be an endometrioma within the dural sac. Endometriosis, therefore, was responsible for the sciatica and subarachnoid hemorrhage [57]. Endometriosis has also been reported to cause muscle masses in the extremities [58].

Neuromuscular Junction

Myasthenia Gravis

Epidemiology

One study of myasthenia gravis found a prevalence rate of 14.2 per 100,000, or approximately 36,000 patients with myasthenia in the United States [59]. In the population less than 50 years old, the condition is 1.5–3.0 times more common in women than men. The incidence rates in males and females over 50 years old are similar. Due to more aggressive treatment and increasing recognition, the average age of patients with myasthenia gravis is gradually increasing.

Pregnancy

Before the modern era, when thymectomy was not commonly used in the management of myasthenia, one-third of patients worsened during pregnancy, one-third remained the same, and one-third improved. It has now been recognized that early thymectomy decreases the risk of clinical deterioration during pregnancy [60]. The course in one pregnancy does not predict the course in another pregnancy. However, most patients will experience a postpartum exacerbation and should be closely monitored in the first month after delivery [38].

Treatment of myasthenia gravis with steroids is not contraindicated in pregnancy. However, azathioprine should be avoided because of its potential teratogenicity. Narcotics should be given cautiously as they decrease respiratory drive. Extra corticosteroids may be required to avoid an addisonian crisis. Labor and delivery are usually normal. Infants should be observed for signs of hypoadrenalism.

Muscle Disorders

Mitochondrial Myopathies

Mitochondrial DNA is maternally inherited. The mitochondrial myopathies include Kearns-Sayre syndrome, mitochondrial encephalopathy with lactic acidosis and stroke (MELAS), and myoclonic epilepsy with ragged red fibers (MERRF).

Patients with Kearns-Sayre syndrome and progressive external ophthalmoplegia have various combinations of progressive ophthalmoplegia, ptosis, pendular nystagmus, heart block, pigmentary retinal degeneration, cerebellar ataxia, pyramidal signs, mild facial and somatic muscle weakness, retarded somatic growth, and raised cerebrospinal fluid (CSF) protein levels [61, 62].

MELAS is a maternally transmitted disease with onset in infancy or childhood. It is characterized by recurrent migraine–like headaches, vomiting, hemiplegia, and hemianopia. Lactic acidosis, ragged red fibers in muscle biopsy specimens, and spongy degeneration of the cortex are the pathologic abnormalities usually identified.

MERRF is a maternally inherited mitochondrial disorder characterized by short stature, myoclonus, nerve deafness, generalized tonic-clonic seizures, ataxia, weakness, and mental and developmental delay with lactic acidosis, spongiform encephalopathy, and the presence of ragged red fibers on muscle biopsy specimens.

Alcoholic Myopathies

Approximately 50% of alcohol abusers have alcoholic muscle disease [63]. It has been demonstrated that female alcohol abusers are at greater risk of myopathy than male alcohol abusers [64].

Inflammatory Myositis

Inflammatory myopathy (polymyositis and dermatomyositis) has a female-to-male incidence ratio of 2.5 to 1.0. This ratio is lower in childhood disease and with associated malignancy, but is very high (10 to 1 female to male) when there is an associated connective tissue disease [65].

Polymyositis and dermatomyositis are generally worsened by pregnancy [66, 67]. Occasional cases begin in pregnancy or the puerperium [68]. Aggressive therapy with corticosteroids is warranted, as 50% of pregnancies with active myositis end in spontaneous abortion or stillbirth. Although fetal intrauterine growth may be retarded, surviving babies thrive after delivery. For these reasons, remission of an active myositis should be achieved before conception if possible.

Dermatomyositis and polymyositis may be associated with gynecologic neoplasms [69] such as ovarian carcinoma [70–72]. There may also be a relationship of polymyositis and dermatomyositis with breast cancer [73].

It has been suggested in the myology literature that there is a specific postmenopausal myopathy. In 1936, Nevin described two cases of late progressive myopathy, which he distinguished from late progressive muscular dystrophy on the basis of the histologic findings of muscle biopsy showing intensive focal segmentary muscle fiber degeneration and phagocytosis without an inflammatory infiltrate [74]. This syndrome has been termed *Nevin's myopathy*. Since then, the debate has raged as to whether Nevin's myopathy is a form of chronic polymyositis, a late muscular dystrophy, or a specific menopausal myopathy [75].

Neuromuscular Complications of Female Malignancies

Neuromuscular complications of neoplasia in women may develop from neural invasion by tumor, as a complication of treatment, or as a paraneoplastic phenomenon.

Direct Effects of Tumors and Complications of Treatment

Radiotherapy to the axilla and the supraclavicular fossa has been commonly used in the treatment of breast carcinoma. One of the recognized late complications of such radiotherapy is a painless plexopathy characterized by myokymic discharges or fasciculations on needle EMG [76, 77]. Possible strategies to avoid this complication include lower doses of radiation or surgical management of the axilla. There appears to be a critical total radiation dose. In one series, 73% of patients who received a 6,300-rad peak dose over 25–26 days developed complications, while only 15% of those at a 5,775-rad dose developed complications [77]. Anticoagulation may be a possible alternative treatment strategy [78, 79].

The differential diagnosis of radiation damage to the brachial plexus in this setting is infiltration of the plexus by malignant tumor. The mean interval from cancer diagnosis to plexopathy tends to be shorter in tumor plexopathy than in radiation plexopathy. Pain is a more prominent feature in tumor plexopathy, whereas women with radiation plexopathy tend to experience paresthesias [76, 80]. Demonstration of a mass with CT or MRI supports a diagnosis of tumor infiltration [81]. Rarely, metastatic breast carcinoma may infiltrate the lumbosacral plexus and produce a painful, progressive lumbosacral plexopathy.

Metastatic breast cancer can produce cranial nerve lesions without intracranial metastases by deposits in the base of skull. Cranial nerves V and VII are the most commonly affected [82]. These lesions are treated with radiation therapy and the average survival time from diagnosis is 20 months.

Metastases from breast carcinoma in the mandible may produce unilateral numbness of the lower lip, chin, and mucous membrane on the inside of the mouth via a mental neuropathy, a condition known as *numb chin syndrome* [83, 84]. A numb chin may even be the presenting sign of the tumor and should initiate a search for cancer.

A postmastectomy pain syndrome occurs after 4–6% of breast operations, especially those involving axillary node dissection. It is caused by interruption of the intercostobrachial nerve and, in some patients, cutaneous branches of other intercostal nerves. Patients experience a constricting, burning sensation and sensory loss in the axilla, posteromedial upper arm, and anterior chest wall. Some prefer the term *postaxillary dissection pain syndrome* as it also occurs in women who have had axillary dissection [85]. Treatment with analgesics, amitriptyline, carbamazepine, and nerve blocks have limited efficacy, but topical capsaicin may be more effective [84].

Radical pelvic surgery for gynecologic cancer may rarely cause nerve injury [86]. The femoral nerve is affected most commonly. Other nerves that may be injured include the sciatic nerve, obturator nerve, genitofemoral nerve, ilioinguinal nerve, iliohypogastric nerve, lateral femoral cutaneous nerve, and pudendal nerve.

Gynecologic cancers may produce lumbosacral plexopathies. Direct invasion by cervical cancer produces lumbosacral plexopathies in 4% of patients [87]. Cervical cancer usually involves the lower plexus (L4–S1). The differential diagnosis may include surgical trauma, spinal metastases, or radiation-induced plexus injury.

Radiation lumbosacral plexopathy may be unilateral at onset but often develops bilaterally later in the course. It tends to be painless. Women that receive less than 4,000 rad are at minimal risk of radiation plexopathy. Tumor patients have unilateral weakness, with pain being the initial symptom and remaining a prominent symptom [88]. EMG and NCS, CT, or MRI may clarify the diagnosis. EMG and NCS may show myokymic discharges in radiation plexopathy and imaging studies may show a mass in neoplastic plexopathy. Radiation treatment has been attempted for neoplastic plexopathy but usually has poor results. The median survival after diagnosis of lumbosacral plexopathy from cervical cancer is 5 months.

Metastatic cervical carcinoma may produce other peripheral nerve problems such as thoracic spinal nerve compression, genitofemoral and obturator nerve compression, and even brachial plexopathy with concomitant Horner's syndrome [89].

Toxic Neuropathies

The neuropathies associated with vincristine [90] and cisplatin [91] are well described in the literature, but a new compound, paclitaxel (Taxol), will be discussed as it is primarily used in ovarian and breast cancer and is associated with a dose-limiting neuropathy.

Taxol has been introduced as a chemotherapeutic agent in platinum-resistant ovarian cancer and in adjuvant chemotherapy of breast cancer. Taxol is a plant alkaloid extracted from the bark of the *Taxus brevifolia,* or western yew tree [92]. It has been a very effective treatment but has a major dose-limiting side effect of neuropathy. An early paper reported a sensory neuropathy [93], and a later paper reported a sensorimotor neuropathy [92]. The threshold for neuropathic side effects appears to be a dose of 200 mg/m^2. Approximately 50% of patients who receive more than 200 mg/m^2 develop a neuropathy. The pathology may be due to a combination of an axonopathy and a neuronopathy [92]. The axonopathy has been demonstrated on sural nerve biopsy [94]. A related compound, docetaxel, causes a similar neuropathy [95].

Paraneoplastic Phenomena

In women with cancer, neurologic abnormalities not caused by the cancer's spread to the nervous system or complications of treatment are paraneoplastic phenomena [96]. Some paraneoplastic complications seen with female malignancies are outlined below.

Women with breast cancer may develop a paraneoplastic peripheral neuropathy involving predominantly sensory fibers or a combination of sensory and motor fibers. The sensory neuropathy presents as often-painful paresthesias involving the hands and the feet, which then progress over a few weeks to involve the entire body and sometimes the face [97]. It has the features of a neuronopathy. All sensory modalities are affected to an equal degree. These patients are often unable to walk due to a severe sensory ataxia. In addition, half of these patients have coexistent involvement of other portions of the nervous system such as limbic encephalitis, subacute cerebellar degeneration, and brain stem encephalitis.

Women with breast cancer may develop a paraneoplastic axonal sensorimotor neuropathy [98]. This disorder progresses very slowly over many years and is not disabling. Most patients remain fully functional as neither the neuropathy nor the breast cancer is disabling.

Paraneoplastic necrotizing myopathy is a rare disorder that has been differentiated from polymyositis [99]. The main features are pain and muscle weakness, predominantly in the proximal shoulder girdle muscles; elevated creatinine kinase levels; and histopathologic signs of muscle necrosis without inflammatory activity. There is no response to corticosteroids. This myopathy has been reported in association with breast carcinoma [100, 101].

Classic textbook teaching has held that peripheral neuropathy caused by necrotizing angiopathy usually appears as a mononeuritis multiplex associated with polyarteritis nodosa or connective tissue diseases such as rheumatoid arthritis or systemic lupus erythematosus [102]. However, mononeuritis multiplex caused by vasculitis may occur as a paraneoplastic syndrome [103]. Paraneoplastic vasculitic neuropathy presenting as mononeuritis multiplex has been reported as a complication of endometrial carcinoma [104]. In one case, a 55-year-old woman with a history of metastatic endometrial carcinoma had asymmetric polyneuropathy, electrophysiologic findings consistent with a diffuse axonal neuropathy, a high sedimentation rate, elevated spinal fluid protein, and microvasculitis with axonal degeneration on nerve biopsy. The patient was treated with 150 mg cyclophosphamide daily with gradual clinical and electrophysiologic improvement.

Small-cell (oat-cell) carcinomas occur predominantly in the lung and are associated with Lambert-Eaton myasthenic syndrome. Small-cell carcinoma also occurs in extrapulmonary locations such as the breast, uterine cervix, and endometrium [105, 106]. Therefore, in a female patient with paraneoplastic Lambert-Eaton myasthenic syndrome without a lung primary tumor, there is the potential for a small-cell carcinoma of uterine origin or a breast carcinoma [106].

The stiff-man syndrome is a rare disease of the central nervous system characterized by rigidity of skeletal muscle. Autoantibodies against glutamic acid decarboxylase are present in 60% of patients with the syndrome. Although the nomenclature may imply otherwise, the condition is well recognized in women. In a subgroup of patients with stiff-man syndrome, the condition may have an autoimmune paraneoplastic origin. A 128-kd autoantibody against a brain protein has been found in three women with stiff-man syndrome. These women were also found to have breast cancer [107].

Acknowledgments

I would like to thank Mrs. E. Meldrum for assistance with the literature search and Dr. G. Stragliotto for linguistic assistance. Supported by the Leslie Eric Paddle Scholarship in the field of Neurology, the Gordon Taylor Scholarship, and the Henry and Rachael Ackman Travelling Scholarship from the University of Melbourne, Australia.

References

1. Alter M. The epidemiology of Guillain-Barré syndrome. Ann Neurol 1990;27:S7.
2. Kuller JA, Katz VL, McCoy C, et al. Pregnancy complicated by Guillain-Barré syndrome. South Med J 1995;88:987.
3. Clifton ER. Guillain-Barré syndrome, pregnancy, and plasmapheresis. J Am Osteopath Assoc 1992;92:1279.
4. Nelson LH, McLean WT. Management of the Landry-Guillain-Barré syndrome in pregnancy. Obstet Gynecol 1985;65:25S.
5. Osterman PO, Fagius J, Lundemo G, et al. Beneficial effects of plasma exchange in acute inflammatory polyradiculoneuropathy. Lancet 1984;2:1296.
6. The Guillain-Barré study group. Plasmapheresis and acute Guillain-Barré syndrome. Neurology 1985;35:1096.
7. Novak DJ, Johnson KP. Relapsing idiopathic polyneuritis during pregnancy. Arch Neurol 1973;28:219.
8. Jones MW, Berry K. Chronic relapsing polyneuritis associated with pregnancy [letter]. Ann Neurol 1981;9:413.
9. McCombe PA, McManis PG, Frith JA, et al. Chronic inflammatory demyelinating polyradiculoneuropathy associated with pregnancy. Ann Neurol 1987;21:102.
10. Calderon-Gonzalez R, Gonzalez-Cantu N, Rizzi-Hernandez H. Recurrent polyneuropathy with pregnancy and oral contraceptives. N Engl J Med 1970;282:1307.
11. Senanayake N, Jeyaratnam J. Toxic polyneuropathy due to gingili oil contaminated with tri-cresyl phosphate affecting adolescent girls in Sri Lanka. Lancet 1981;1:88.
12. Schipper HM. Neurology of sex steriods and oral contraceptives. Neurol Clin 1986;4:721.
13. Tschudy D, Valsamis M, Magnussen C. Acute intermittent porphyria: clinical and selected research aspects. Ann Intern Med 1975;83:851.

14. Lamon JM, Frykholm BC, Herrera W, et al. Danazol administration to females with menses-associated exacerbations of acute intermittent porphyria. J Clin Endocrinol Metab 1979;48:123.
15. Anonymous. The pill and porphyria. BMJ 1972;3:603.
16. Anderson KE, Spitz IM, Sassa S, et al. Prevention of cyclical attacks of acute intermittent porphyria with a long-acting agonist of luteinizing hormone-releasing hormone. N Engl J Med 1984;311:643.
17. Adour KK, Wingred J. Idiopathic facial paralysis (Bell's palsy): factors affecting severity and outcome in 446 patients. Neurology 1974;24:1112.
18. Hilsinger RL, Adour KK, Doty HE. Idiopathic facial paralysis, pregnancy and the menstrual cycle. Ann Otol Rhinol Laryngol 1975;84:433.
19. Gbolade BA. Recurrent lower motor neurone facial paralysis in four successive pregnancies. J Laryngol Otol 1994;108:587.
20. Phalen GS. Reflections on 21 years experience with the carpal tunnel syndrome. JAMA 1970;212:1365.
21. Kimura J. Electrodiagnosis in Diseases of Nerve and Muscle: Principles and Practice (2nd ed). Philadelphia: FA Davis, 1989.
22. Radecki P. A gender specific wrist ratio and the likelihood of a median nerve abnormality at the carpal tunnel. Am J Phys Med Rehabil 1994;73:157.
23. Dekel S, Coates R. Primary carpal stenosis as a cause of "idiopathic" carpal-tunnel syndrome. Lancet 1979;2:1024.
24. Dawson DM, Hallett M, Millender LH. Entrapment Neuropathies. Boston: Little, Brown, 1983.
25. Wand JS. Carpal tunnel syndrome in pregnancy and lactation. J Hand Surg [Br] 1990;15:93.
26. Stahl S, Blumenfeld Z, Yarnitsky D. Carpal tunnel syndrome in pregnancy: indications for early surgery. J Neurol Sci 1996;136:182.
27. Wand JS. The natural history of carpal tunnel syndrome in lactation. J R Soc Med 1989;82:349.
28. Sabour M, Fadel H. The carpal tunnel syndrome: a new complication ascribed to the "pill." Am J Obstet Gynecol 1970;107:1265.
29. Parsonage MJ, Turner JWA. Neuralgic amyotrophy: the shoulder-girdle syndrome. Lancet 1948;1:973.
30. Taylor RA. Heredofamilial mononeuritis multiplex with brachial predilection. Brain 1960;83:113.
31. Bradley WG, Madrid R, Thrush DC, et al. Recurrent brachial plexus neuropathy. Brain 1975;98:381.
32. Redmond JMT, Cros D, Martin JB, et al. Relapsing bilateral brachial plexopathy during pregnancy. Arch Neurol 1989;46:462.
33. Lederman RJ, Wilborn AJ. Postpartum neuralgic amyotrophy [abstract]. Neurology 1993;43:A190.
34. Simkin P. Intermittent brachial plexus neuropathy secondary to breast engorgement. Birth 1988;15:102.
35. Hueston WJ, Locke KT. Norplant neuropathy: peripheral neurologic symptoms associated with subdermal contraceptive implants. J Fam Pract 1995;40:184.

36. LaBan MM, Perrin JCS, Latimer FR. Pregnancy and the herniated lumbar disc. Arch Phys Med Rehabil 1983;64:319.
37. Kelsey JL, Greenberg RA, Hardy RJ, et al. Pregnancy and the syndrome of the herniated lumbar intervertebral disc: an epidemiological study. Yale J Biol Med 1975;48:361.
38. Rosenbaum RB, Donaldson JO. Peripheral nerve and neuromuscular disorders. Neurol Clin 1994;12:461.
39. Hakim MA, Katirji MB. Femoral mononeuropathy induced by the lithotomy position: a report of 5 cases with a review of the literature. Muscle Nerve 1993;16:891.
40. Carter BL, Racz GB. Iliohypogastric nerve entrapment in pregnancy: diagnosis and treatment. Anesth Analg 1994;79:1193.
41. Enkin MW. Commentary: entrapment neuropathies in birth and breastfeeding. Birth 1988;5:104.
42. Colachis SC, Pease WS, Johnson EW. A preventable cause of foot drop during childbirth. Am J Obstet Gynecol 1994;171:270.
43. Reif ME. Bilateral common peroneal nerve palsy secondary to prolonged squatting in natural childbirth. Birth 1988;15:100.
44. Kane RE. Neurologic deficits following epidural or spinal anesthesia. Anesth Analg 1981;60:150.
45. Yuen EC, Layzer RB, Weitz SR, et al. Neurologic complications of lumbar epidural anesthesia and analgesia. Neurology 1995;45:1795.
46. Swash M, Snooks SJ, Henry MM. Unifying concept of pelvic floor disorders and incontinence. J R Soc Med 1985;78:906.
47. Thind P, Lose G. The effect of bilateral pudendal blockade in the static urethral closing function in healthy females. Obstet Gynecol 1992;80:906.
48. Snooks SJ, Swash M. Perineal nerve and transcutaneous spinal stimulation: new methods for investigation of the urethral striated sphincter musculature. Br J Urol 1984;56:406.
49. Sultan SJ, Kamm MA, Hudson CN. Pudendal nerve damage during labour: prospective study before and after childbirth. Br J Obstet Gynecol 1994;101:22.
50. Tetzschner T, Sorensen M, Rasmussen OO, et al. Pudendal nerve damage increases the risk of fecal incontinence in women with anal sphincter rupture after childbirth. Acta Obstet Gynecol Scand 1995;74:434.
51. Salazar-Grueso E, Roos R. Sciatic endometriosis: a treatable sensorimotor mononeuropathy. Neurology 1986;36:1360.
52. Richards BJ, Gillett WR, Pollock M. Reversal of foot drop in sciatic nerve endometriosis [letter]. J Neurol Neurosurg Psychiatry 1991;54:935.
53. Cottier JP, Descamps P, Sonier CB, et al. Sciatic endometriosis: MR evaluation. AJNR Am J Neuroradiol 1995;16:1399.
54. Head HB, Welch JS, Mussey E, et al. Cyclic sciatica: report of a case with a new surgical sign. JAMA 1962;180:521.
55. DeCesare SL, Yeko TR. Sciatic nerve endometriosis treated with a gonadotropin releasing hormone agonist. J Reprod Med 1995;40:226.

56. Fischer S. Seltene lokalisation einer Endometriosis externa extraperitonealis. Geburtshilfe Frauenheilkd 1953;13:240.
57. Lombardo L, Mateos JH, Barroeta FF. Subarachnoid hemorrhage due to endometriosis of the spinal canal. Neurology 1968;18:423.
58. Duncan C, Pitney WR. Endometrial tumours in the extremities. Med J Aust 1949;2:715.
59. Phillips LH. The epidemiology of myasthenia gravis. Neurol Clin 1994;12:263.
60. Eden RD, Gall SA. Myasthenia gravis and pregnancy: a reappraisal of thymectomy. Obstet Gynecol 1983;62:328.
61. Pryse-Phillips W. Companion to Clinical Neurology. Boston: Little, Brown, 1995.
62. Johns DR. Mitochondrial DNA and disease. N Engl J Med 1995;333:638.
63. Preedy VR, Salisbury JR, Peters TJ. Alcoholic muscle disease: features and mechanisms. J Pathol 1994;173:309.
64. Urbano-Marquez A, Estruch R, Fernadez-Sola J, et al. The greater risk of alcoholic cardiomyopathy and myopathy in women compared with men. JAMA 1995;274:149.
65. Medsger TA, Oddis CV. Inflammatory Muscle Disease. In JH Klippel, PA Dieppe (eds), Rheumatology. St. Louis: Mosby, 1994.
66. Houck W, Melnyk C, Gast MJ. Polymyositis in pregnancy, a case report and literature review. J Reprod Med 1987;32:208.
67. King CR, Chow S. Dermatomyositis and pregnancy. Obstet Gynecol 1985;66:589.
68. Steiner I, Averbuch-Heller L, Abramsky O, et al. Postpartum idiopathic polymyositis. Lancet 1992;339:256.
69. Antel JP, Moumdjian R. Paraneoplastic syndromes: a role for the immune system. J Neurol 1989;236:1.
70. Hudson CN, Curling M, Potsides P, et al. Paraneoplastic syndromes in patients with ovarian neoplasia. J R Soc Med 1993;86:202.
71. Armes JE, Rome R, Ostor AG, et al. A case of polymyositis and invasive squamous cell carcinoma of the uterine cervix. Aust N Z J Obstet Gynaecol 1993;33:440.
72. Peters WA, Andersen WA, Thornton, WN. Dermatomyositis and coexistent ovarian cancer: a review of the compounding clinical problems. Gynecol Oncol 1983;15:440.
73. Sigurgeirsson B, Lindelof B, Edhag O, et al. Risk of cancer in patients with dermatomyositis and polymyositis. A population based study. N Engl J Med 1992;326:363.
74. Bekeny G, Benke B, Toro I, et al. A case of late myopathy of polymyositic origin. Report of biopsy. Acta Neuropathol 1967;9:53.
75. Bagnoli P, Zocchi G. Sulla miopatia della menopausa detta di Nevin. Minerva Ginecol 1979;31:205.
76. Lederman RJ, Wilbourn AJ. Brachial plexopathy: recurrent cancer or radiation? Neurology 1984;34:1331.

77. Stoll RA, Andrews JT. Radiation-induced peripheral neuropathy. BMJ 1966;1:834.
78. Glantz MJ, Burger PC, Friedman AH, et al. Treatment of radiation-induced nervous system injury with heparin and warfarin. Neurology 1994;44:2020.
79. Koehler PJ, Jager J, Verbiest H, et al. Anticoagulation for radiation injury [letter]. Neurology 1995;45:1786.
80. Harper CM, Thomas JE, Cascino TL, et al. Distinction between neoplastic and radiation-induced brachial plexopathy, with emphasis on the role of EMG. Neurology 1989;39:502.
81. Thyagarajan D, Cascino T, Harms G. Magnetic resonance imaging in brachial plexopathy of cancer. Neurology 1995;45:421.
82. Hall SM, Buzdar AU, Blumenschein GR. Cranial nerve palsies in metastatic breast cancer due to osseous metastasis without intracranial involvement. Cancer 1983;52:180.
83. Massey EW, Moore J, Schold SC. Mental neuropathy from systemic cancer. Neurology 1981;31:1277.
84. Anderson KE, Spitz IM, Sassa S, et al. Prevention of cyclical attacks of acute intermittent porphyria with a long-acting agonist of luteinizing hormone-releasing hormone. N Engl J Med 1984;311:643.
85. Vecht CJ, Van de Brand HJ, Wajer OJ. Post-axillary dissection pain in breast cancer due to a lesion of the intercostobrachial nerve. Pain 1989;38:171.
86. Hoffman MS, Roberts WS, Cavanagh D. Neuropathies associated with radical pelvic surgery for gynecologic cancer. Gynecol Oncol 1988;31:462.
87. Fadul CE. Neurological Complications of Genitourinary Cancer. In RG Wiley (ed), Neurological Complications of Cancer. New York: Marcel Dekker, 1995.
88. Thomas JE, Cascino TL, Earle JD. Differential diagnosis between radiation and tumor plexopathy of the pelvis. Neurology 1985;35:1.
89. Saphner T, Gallion HH, Van Nagell JR, et al. Neurologic complications of cervical carcinoma. A review of 2261 cases. Cancer 1989;64:1147.
90. Casey EB, Jellife AM, Le Quesne PA, et al. Vincristine neuropathy. Clinical and electrophysiological observations. Brain 1973;96:69.
91. Boogerd W, Huinink WWB, Dalesio O, et al. Cisplatin induced neuropathy: central, peripheral and autonomic nerve involvement. J Neurooncol 1990;9:255.
92. Chaudhry V, Rowinsky EK, Sartorius SE, et al. Peripheral neuropathy from Taxol and cisplatin combination chemotherapy: clinical and electrophysiological studies. Ann Neurol 1994;35:304.
93. Lipton RB, Apfel SC, Dutcher JP, et al. Taxol produces a predominantly sensory neuropathy. Neurology 1989;39:368.
94. Sahenk Z, Barohn R, New P, et al. Taxol neuropathy. Electrodiagnostic and sural nerve biopsy findings. Arch Neurol 1994;51:726.
95. Hilkens PHE, Verweij J, Stoter G, et al. Peripheral neurotoxicity induced by docetaxel. Neurology 1996;46:104.
96. Posner JB. Neurologic Complications of Cancer. Philadelphia: FA Davis, 1995.

97. Moots PL. Peripheral Nervous System Complications in Cancer Patients. In RG Wiley (ed), Neurological Complications of Cancer. New York: Marcel Dekker, 1995.
98. Peterson K, Forsyth PA, Posner JB. Paraneoplastic sensorimotor neuropathy associated with breast cancer. J Neurooncol 1994;21:159.
99. Vobkamper M, Korf B, Franke F, et al. Paraneoplastic necrotizing myopathy: a rare disorder to be differentiated from polymyositis. J Neurol 1989;236:489.
100. Urich H, Wilkinson M. Necrosis of muscle with carcinoma: myositis or myopathy? J Neurol Neurosurg Psychiatry 1970;33:398.
101. Smith B. Skeletal muscle necrosis associated with cancer. J Pathol 1969;97:207.
102. Kissel JT, Slivka AP, Warmolts JR, et al. The clinical spectrum of necrotizing angiopathy of the peripheral nervous system. Ann Neurol 1985;18:251.
103. Johnson PC, Rolak LA, Hamilton RH, et al. Paraneoplastic vasculitis of nerve: a remote effect of cancer. Ann Neurol 1979;5:437.
104. Oh SJ, Slaughter R, Harrell L. Paraneoplastic vasculitic neuropathy: a treatable neuropathy. Muscle Nerve 1991;14:152.
105. Ibrahim NBM, Briggs JC, Corbishley CM. Extrapulmonary oat-cell carcinoma. Cancer 1984;54:1645.
106. O'Neill JH, Murray NM, Newsom-Davis J. The Lambert-Eaton myasthenic syndrome. A review of 50 cases. Brain 1988;111:577.
107. Folli F, Solimena M, Cofiell R, et al. Autoantibodies to a 128-kd synaptic protein in three women with the stiff-man syndrome and breast cancer. N Engl J Med 1993;328:546.

CHAPTER 7

Cognition and Alzheimer's Disease

Michael C. Irizarry, Teresa Gómez-Isla,
and Bradley T. Hyman

Alzheimer's disease (AD) exacts a heavy emotional, physical, and financial toll from patients and their families and places a significant economic burden on society. Prevalence rates for dementia, commonly caused by AD, are 3.4–7.8% of people aged 65 years and older, increasing with age to 23–28% of those aged 85 years or older [1]. In the United States, the economic costs of caring for over 3.75 million affected individuals reflect estimated annual direct and indirect costs of care for each patient of up to $47,000 per year [2]. Women are disproportionately affected compared to men, with female-to-male prevalence ratios as high as 2.8 to 1.0 for AD in the Framingham cohort [3]. Treatments to reduce the risk of AD or its severity would thus be of tremendous benefit, and the use of estrogen replacement therapy in postmenopausal women has been suggested as one such treatment. This chapter reviews the effects of estrogen on cognition, AD risk, and AD symptomatology. Gender differences in cognitive function and AD clinical features are also considered.

Gender Differences in Cognitive Function

Males and females do not differ in general intelligence and overall neuropsychological function, as evidenced by full-scale Wechsler Adult Intelligence Scale (WAIS), Intelligence Quotient, and Halstead-Reitan Battery (HRB) summary scores in a study of 177 males and 177 females matched for age and education [4]. On individual tests within this battery, males performed statistically significantly better in tests of motor speed (finger-tapping test), grip strength (hand dynamometer), and the tactual performance test-total time, while females performed significantly better in the aphasia screening exam and the WAIS comprehension subtest [4]. These results support the impression, based on neuropsychological test performance, that sex differences exist in specific cognitive domains. On average, men appear to perform better in spatial, quantitative, and gross motor strength testing, while women perform better in verbal skills, perceptual ability, and fine motor testing, with differences in the range of 0.25–1.00 standard deviation [4, 5]. Differential effects of gender on age-related changes in immediate recall of designs, short-term visual memory, visual perception, and visual construction ability were evaluated by the Benton Visual Retention Test (BVRT) in 673 nondemented participants in the Baltimore Longitudinal Study of Aging [6]. Cross-section analysis did not reveal a sex difference in overall BVRT performance, although the pattern of impairment differed, with females exhibiting statistically significant greater omission and rotation errors than males. Longitudinal analysis showed that males, however, had a steeper increase in omission errors with age. The greater rotation errors in females are consistent with better performance by males in tests of spatial rotation ability; nonetheless, the gender differences accounted for less than 1% of the variance in BVRT error profiles [6]. Menstrual cycle–related changes in cognitive functioning have been described, with spatial skills inversely related and verbal skills directly related to high estrogen states [5].

Effects of Estrogen on Cognitive Function

The role of estrogen in modulating cognition and behavior is supported by basic research studies. Estrogen increases the activity of choline acetyltransferase [7] and promotes neurite outgrowth in cholinergic neurons [8]. Effects of estrogen replacement in ovariectomized or senescent rats include preserving dendritic spine density in CA1 hippocampal neurons after ovariectomy [9], enhancing brain glucose utilization [10], and improving sensorimotor behavior [11, 12].

Estrogen replacement therapy has been associated with improvements in mood and behavior in postmenopausal women. A double-blind study of 28 elderly postmenopausal female residents in a home for the elderly, with 12 randomized to 0.625 mg of Premarin and 16 to placebo, found that the group receiving estrogen demonstrated significant and progressive improvement in psychological questionnaire scores in the categories of communication and interpersonal relations and care of self and social responsibility, while the scores of the placebo group declined in these areas over a 1-year period. The study was limited by the high dropout rate of the initial 50 women randomized [13]. A randomized, placebo-controlled, double-blind prospective study of Premarin, 0.625 and 1.25 mg per day, in 36 postmenopausal ovariectomized women demonstrated that estrogen improved mood and subjective measures of memory. Significant improvement with estrogen therapy was noted in the Beck Depression Inventory and income management scores in the Profile of Adaptation to Life. No significant effect was seen on the WAIS digit span and digit symbol, which are tests of executive and short-term memory processes, or on the Minnesota Multiphasic Personality Inventory [14].

Estrogen may have beneficial effects on memory independent of effects on mood. A neuropsychological study of 31 women before and 3 months after hysterectomy with salpingo-oophorectomy randomized to postoperative placebo or monthly 10 mg intramuscular estradiol valerate showed statistically significant preservation of immediate and delayed recall of paired associations (as tested by the Wechsler Memory Scale) correlated with blood estrone and estradiol levels, relative to a decline in these scores in the placebo group. The treated group also showed improvement in immediate paragraph recall relative to preoperative performance, with no change in the placebo group. No difference among treated groups in pre- and postoperative scores were noted in delayed paragraph recall, visual reproduction, digit span, or mood measures by the Multiple Affect Adjective Check List [15]. A retrospective case-control study of 72 cognitively intact postmenopausal women taking estrogen matched with a group not taking estrogen showed significantly higher scores in the group taking estrogen on a proper name recall task but not on a word recall test [16]. Another study found that compared to 43 postmenopausal women not taking estrogen, 28 postmenopausal women on estrogen replacement therapy scored higher in tests of immediate paragraph recall and delayed paragraph recall; the groups did not differ in immediate or delayed paired associates and selective reminding tests, or in tests of language, spatial memory, spatial skills, and attention [17]. These results, as well as those of other studies, support the idea that estrogen does affect cognitive ability [18–20]. This effect seems more pronounced in verbal memory function than in visual recall.

Several other studies do not confirm this effect of estrogen on memory [14, 21, 22]. A large cross-sectional epidemiologic study of 800 women aged 65–95 found no consistent association between estrogen use and cognitive function measured by the Buschke-Fuld Selective Reminding Test, Visual Reproduction Test (Wechsler Memory Scale), Mini-Mental State Examination (MMSE), Blessed Information-Memory-Concentration Test, Trails B (from the HRB), and category fluency [23]. Factors possibly contributing to the conflicting results among these studies include estrogen formulation, duration of treatment, specific cognitive tests performed, and lack of evaluation of hormonal status through determinations of circulating hormone levels [5]. These putative effects of estrogen on cognitive function have led to studies examining the role of estrogen in the risk and treatment of AD.

Gender Differences in Alzheimer's Disease Risk and Clinical Course

Most epidemiologic studies demonstrate sex differences in AD risk [24], and some suggest that female gender is an independent risk factor for AD [25]. Females are more likely to develop AD, in part because they have a longer life expectancy than men. The prevalence is greater in females, with female-to-male prevalence ratios ranging from 1.2:1.0 to 2.8:1.0 in American populations [1, 3], although it is unclear if this prevalence actually reflects an increased incidence in females [26]. Also, some case-control and population-based studies show a gender interaction with the risk for AD and cognitive impairment conferred by the apolipoprotein E (apoE) ε4 allele, with apoE ε4 having a greater impact on cognitive decline in women than in men [27–29].

Some clinical features of AD also show gender-based differences. The mean age of onset is older in females [30], and women with the disease have a longer time of survival after the onset of disease [30, 31]. Disease course, however, is not significantly affected by gender. Rate of decline in most cognitive tests does not differ between males and females [32, 33]. Furthermore, rate of progression of neuropathologic features of AD such as neuronal loss and the development of neurofibrillary tangles is identical in women and men (Figures 7.1 and 7.2) [34].

Although the clinical course of AD is similar in men and women, the extent of cognitive deficits as determined by neuropsychological testing appears to show statistically significant gender differences, particularly in tests of language function. A study of 22 men and 24 women with probable AD who were matched for age, education, age of onset, and duration of symptoms showed that women performed worse on the Boston Naming Test and a test of praxis. Males and females performed similarly on a visuospatial task, narrative writing task, and the Orientation-Memory-Concentration Test modified from the Blessed. These studies were extended to a Consortium to Establish a Registry for Alzheimer's Disease database of 270 men and 377 women with probable AD. Analysis controlling for age, education, and dementia duration found significant gender effects, with women performing more poorly on a naming task (from the Boston Naming Test), verbal fluency, rate of forgetting, and delayed recall of previously rehearsed word names; however, visuospatial function and immediate recall were equally impaired in men and women. These significant differences were relatively small, with less than 4% of the total variance on the neuropsychological tests due to gender [35]. An Italian sample of 22 men and 30 women with mild AD found women to be significantly more impaired in the Boston Naming Test and the information subtest of the WAIS, with no difference in impairment in verbal fluency, Stroop test, logical memory, and verbal list learning [36]. A longitudinal study of 29 men and 31 women with probable AD who were matched for age, education,

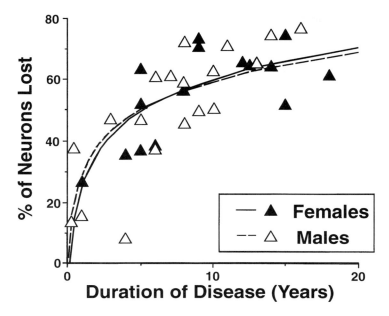

FIGURE 7.1. The percentage of neurons lost relative to the average number in nondemented controls in the superior temporal sulcus of 15 female and 19 male Alzheimer's disease patients correlates with the duration of illness independent of gender [34].

and MMSE score confirmed poorer performance by women in the Boston Naming Test, with equal impairment between men and women in word fluency, Token Test, and Reporter's Test. Over 18 months, the differences in Boston Naming Test persisted, but the rate of decline in all tests was not different between men and women [33]. Thus, collectively, women with AD consistently appear to perform worse in language function as reflected by the Boston Naming Test.

Estrogen and Alzheimer's Disease

The studies of estrogen effects on memory have been extended to patients with AD, in which estrogen may have both a preventative and a cognitive-enhancing effect. Epidemiologic studies suggest that postmenopausal estrogen use is associated with a reduced risk of AD. A preventative effect of oral estrogen was concluded by a retrospective case-control comparison of 235 elderly women volunteers with either probable AD or no cognitive impairment [37]. Estrogens were used by 17 (18%) of the 92 nondemented controls compared to 10 (7%) of the 143 AD cases, yielding a relative risk

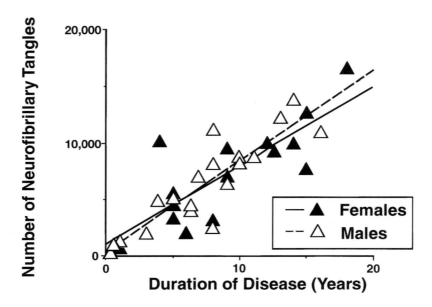

FIGURE 7.2.   Total neurofibrillary tangles in a 700 μm–wide region of the superior temporal sulcus correlates with duration of illness independent of gender in 15 female and 19 male Alzheimer's disease patients [34].

(RR) of AD with estrogen treatment of 0.33 (95% CI 0.15–0.74) compared to no treatment with estrogen [38]. The AD patients taking estrogen also performed better on the MMSE than AD patients not taking estrogen. The study was limited by reliance on primary caregivers for information on estrogen-use history of the AD patients and because the study was not population based [37]. From a prospectively followed cohort that enrolled 8,877 women in a California retirement community, 138 women with a diagnosis of AD or related dementia on death certificates were age-matched with 552 women with other causes of death. A lower incidence of AD on death certificates was found in estrogen users (RR 0.69; 95% CI 0.46–1.03) versus nonusers, with the risk decreasing with increasing estrogen dose (RR 0.46; 95% CI 0.22–0.94 with ≥1.25 mg/day estrogen) and duration of therapy (RR 0.49; 95% CI 0.27–0.88 with ≥7 years of treatment). In this study, estrogen use was assessed by a survey given at the time of recruitment and periodically afterward during the longitudinal study [39]. A case-control study of 107 female AD patients and 120 age-matched female controls enrolled in a Seattle health maintenance organization did not find a significant association between estrogen exposure (as determined by pharmacy records) and the risk of AD (RR of AD with estrogen exposure 1.1; 95% CI 0.6–1.8); RRs were reduced with oral estrogen exposure alone (RR 0.7; 95% CI 0.4–1.5), prolonged use (RR 0.8; 95% CI 0.3–1.8), and current use (RR 0.6; 95% CI 0.3–1.2) [40].

Two recent large prospective studies provide strong evidence for a protective effect of estrogen. Thirty-eight of 514 postmenopausal and peri-menopausal women followed prospectively in the Baltimore Longitudinal Study of Aging developed AD; the relative risk for AD in estrogen users (as documented prospectively in each study visit) versus nonusers was 0.44 (95% CI 0.20–0.97), adjusted for education level [41, 42]. A relative risk of AD with estrogen use of 0.40 (95% CI 0.22–0.85) was found in 1,124 cognitively intact postmenopausal women (aged 74.2 ± 1.7 years) followed longitudinally for 1–5 years in northern Manhattan, New York City. This corresponded to an annual AD incidence rate of 2.7% in the women taking estrogen compared to 8.4% in those not taking estrogen. Estrogen use was associated with younger age, more years of education, hysterectomy, earlier age of menopause, white or Hispanic ethnicity, lowered risk of AD, and delayed age of onset of AD. Adjustment for ethnic group, education, and apoE genotype did not significantly change this relative risk [43]. Thus, most prospective case-control and population-based studies have found a reduced risk of AD with oral estrogen replacement therapy; however, only the confidence intervals of the more recent longitudinal studies are significant, and the extent of the protective effect is unclear.

Cognitive effects of estrogen in AD treatment have been evaluated in small preliminary studies. An open label study of estradiol, 2 mg per day, found that three of seven women with AD showed improvement over 6 weeks measured against baseline psychometric testing on the MMSE, Hamilton Depression Scale, and Randt Memory Test. Those who responded to the therapy tended to be older, with milder dementia, affective symptoms, osteoporosis, and lower baseline serum estrogen levels [44]. Another unblinded study showed improvement in dementia screening tests over 6 weeks in six of seven patients treated with Premarin, 1.25 mg per day, particularly in measures of memory, orientation, and concentration [45]. Fifteen AD patients treated with Premarin, 1.25 mg per day for 6 weeks, demonstrated improvements in the group mean MMSE, Hasegawa Dementia Scale, and regional right frontal blood flow by single photon emission computed tomography [46]. An improvement in the mean MMSE was seen in 10 women with AD treated with 0.625 mg per day of Premarin over 5 months [47]. A double-blind, placebo-controlled trial of Premarin, 1.25 mg per day for 3 weeks, showed statistically significant improvement in the mean MMSE of the seven women receiving estrogen, while there was no change in the mean MMSE scores of the seven receiving placebo [48]. These reports suggest that estrogen may be effective in improving memory, orientation, and calculation in women with mild to moderate dementia [38]. Large clinical studies are in progress to assess prospectively the response of AD to estrogen treatment [49] and the risk of cognitive decline in postmenopausal women with estrogen replacement therapy [50].

Estrogen therapy may also enhance responsiveness to cholinergic therapy in AD. Using post-hoc analysis, women taking estrogen and tacrine (Cognex) were found to perform significantly better than women on placebo or tacrine alone on the outcome measures of the Alzheimer's Disease Assessment Scale—Cognitive Scale, Clinician's Interview-Based Impression of Change, MMSE, and Caregiver's Impression of Change [51].

Conclusion

Mild sex differences in cognitive function have been observed in specific cognitive domains, with males performing better in spatial tasks and females in verbal skills. In AD, the female advantage in verbal skills disappears, as women with AD perform more poorly on neuropsychological tests of language function. The beneficial effects of estrogen replacement therapy on mood and cognition in postmenopausal women have led to studies of estrogen, AD risk, and AD symptoms. Epidemiologic studies suggest that estrogen has a protective effect in reducing the risk for AD, and clinical studies demonstrate a cognition-enhancing effect of estrogen in a subset of AD patients. Larger epidemiologic and clinical studies will attempt to confirm these benefits attributed to estrogen replacement therapy.

References

1. Beard CM, Kokmen E, O'Brien PC, et al. The prevalence of dementia is changing over time in Rochester, Minnesota. Neurology 1995;45:75.
2. Max W. The economic impact of Alzheimer's disease. Neurology 1993;43(Suppl 14):S6.
3. Bachman DL, Wolf PA, Linn R, et al. Prevalence of dementia and probable senile dementia of the Alzheimer type in the Framingham Study. Neurology 1992;42:115.
4. Heaton RK, Grant I, Matthews CG. Differences in Neuropsychological Test Performance Associated with Age, Education, and Sex. In I Grant, KM Adams (eds), Neuropsychological Assessment of Neuropsychiatric Disorders. New York: Oxford University Press, 1986;100.
5. Sherwin BB. Estrogenic effects on memory in women. Ann N Y Acad Sci 1994;743:213.
6. Resnick SM, Trotman K, Kawas C, et al. Age-associated changes in specific errors on the Benton Visual Retention Test. J Gerontol B Psychol Sci Soc Sci 1995;50:171.
7. Liune VN. Estradiol increases choline acetyltransferase activity in specific basal forebrain nuclei and projection areas of female rats. Exp Neurol 1985;89:484.

8. Honjo H, Tamura T, Matsumoto Y, et al. Estrogen as a growth factor to central nervous cells. J Steroid Biochem Mol Bio 1992;41:633.

9. Gould E, Woolly CS, Frankfurt M, et al. Gonadal steroids regulate dendritic spine density in hippocampal pyramidal cells in adulthood. J Neurosci 1990;10:1286.

10. Namba H, Solokoff L. Acute brain administration of high doses of estrogen increases glucose utilization throughout the brain. Brain Res 1984;291:391.

11. Joseph JA, Kochman K, Roth GS. Reduction of motor behavioral deficits in senescence via chronic prolactin or estrogen administration: time course and putative mechanisms of action. Brain Res 1989;505:195.

12. McDermott JL, Kreutzberg JD, Liu B, et al. Effects of estrogen treatment on sensorimotor task performance and brain dopamine concentrations in gonadectomized male and female CD-1 mice. Horm Behav 1994;28:16.

13. Kantor HI, Michael CM, Shore H, et al. Administration of estrogens to older women, a psychometric evaluation. Am J Obstet Gynecol 1968;101:658.

14. Ditkoff EC, Crary WG, Cristo M, et al. Estrogen improves psychological function in asymptomatic postmenopausal women. Obstet Gynecol 1991;78:991.

15. Phillips SM Sherwin BB. Effects of estrogen on memory function in surgically menopausal women. Psychoneuroendocrinology 1992;17:485.

16. Robinson D, Friedman L, Marcus R, et al. Estrogen replacement therapy and memory in older women. J Am Geriatr Soc 1994;42:919.

17. Kampen DL, Sherwin BB. Estrogen use and verbal memory in healthy postmenopausal women. Obstet Gynecol 1994;83:979.

18. Hackman BW, Galbraith D. Six month study of oestrogen therapy with piperazine oestrone sulphate and its effect on memory. Curr Med Res Opin 1977;4(Suppl):21.

19. Sherwin BB. Estrogen and/or androgen replacement therapy and cognitive functioning in surgically menopausal women. Psychoneuroendocrinology 1988;13:345.

20. Caldwell BM, Watson RL. An evaluation of psychologic effects of sex hormone administration in aged women. Results of therapy after six months. J Gerontol 1952;7:228.

21. Rauramo L, Langerspetz K, Engblom P, et al. The effect of castration and peroral estrogen therapy on some psychological functions. Front Horm Res 1975;8:133.

22. Vanhulle G, Demol R. A Double-Blind Study into the Influence of Estriol on a Number of Psychological Tests in Post-Menopausal Women. In PA van Keep, RB Greenblatt, M Albeaux-Fernet (eds), Consensus on Menopausal Research. Lancaster, England: MTP Press, 1976;94.

23. Barrett-Connor E, Kritz-Silverstein D. Estrogen replacement therapy and cognitive function in older women. JAMA 1993;269:2637.

24. Katzman R, Kawas C. The Epidemiology of Dementia and Alzheimer Disease. In RD Terry, R Katzman, KL Bick (eds), Alzheimer Disease. New York: Raven, 1994;105.

25. Rocca WA, Bonaiuto S, Lippi A, et al. Prevalence of clinically diagnosed Alzheimer's disease and other dementing disorders: a door-to-door survey in Appignano, Macerata Province, Italy. Neurology 1990;40:626.
26. Kokmen E, Beard CM, O'Brien PC, et al. Is the incidence of dementing illness changing: a 25-year trend study in Rochester, Minnesota (1960–1984). Neurology 1993;43:1887.
27. Payami H, Montee K, Kaye J, et al. Alzheimer's disease, apolipoprotein E and gender. JAMA 1994;271:1316.
28. Hyman BT, Gómez-Isla T, Briggs M, et al. Apolipoprotein E and cognitive change in an elderly population. Ann Neurol 1996;40:55.
29. Gómez-Isla T, West HL, Rebeck GW, et al. Clinical and pathological correlates of apolipoprotein E ε4 in Alzheimer's disease. Ann Neurol 1996;39:62.
30. Kokmen E, Beard CM, O'Brien PC, et al. Epidemiology of dementia in Rochester, Minnesota. Mayo Clin Proc 1996;71:272.
31. Beard CM, Kokmen E, O'Brien PC, et al. Are patients with Alzheimer's disease surviving longer in recent years? Neurology 1994;44:1869.
32. Locasio JJ, Growdon JH, Corkin S. Cognitive test performance in detecting, staging, and tracking Alzheimer's disease. Arch Neurol 1995;52:1087.
33. Ripich DN, Petrill SA, Whitehouse PJ, et al. Gender differences in language of AD patients: a longitudinal study. Neurology 1995;45:299.
34. Gómez-Isla T, Hollister R, West H, et al. Neuronal loss correlates with but exceeds neurofibrillary tangles in Alzheimer's disease. Ann Neurol 1996 (in press).
35. Henderson VW, Buckwalter JG. Cognitive deficits of men and women with Alzheimer's disease. Neurology 1994;44:90.
36. Padovani A, Magni E, Cappa S, et al. Language, Alzheimer's disease, and gender. Neurology 1996;46:592.
37. Henderson VW, Paganini-Hill A, Emanuel CK, et al. Estrogen replacement therapy in older women: comparisons between Alzheimer's disease cases and nondemented control subjects. Arch Neurol 1994;51:896.
38. Paganini-Hill A. Oestrogen replacement therapy and Alzheimer's disease. Br J Obstet Gynaecol 1996;103(Suppl 13):80.
39. Paganini-Hill A, Henderson VW. Estrogen deficiency and risk of Alzheimer's disease in women. Am J Epidemiol 1994;140:256.
40. Brenner DE, Kukull WA, Stergachis A, et al. Postmenopausal estrogen replacement therapy and the risk of Alzheimer's disease: a population-based case-control study. Am J Epidemiol 1994;140:262.
41. Morrison A, Resnick S, Corrada M, et al. A prospective study of estrogen replacement therapy and the risk of developing Alzheimer's disease in the Baltimore Longitudinal Study of Aging. Neurology 1996;46:A435.
42. Stephensen J. More evidence links NSAID, estrogen use with reduced Alzheimer risk. JAMA 1996;275:1389.
43. Tang M-X, Jacobs D, Stern Y, et al. Effect of oestrogen during menopause on risk and age at onset of Alzheimer's disease. Lancet 1996;348:429.

44. Fillit H, Weinreb H, Cholst I, et al. Observations in a preliminary open trial of estradiol therapy for senile dementia-Alzheimer's type. Psychoneuroendocrinology 1986;11:337.

45. Honjo H, Ogino Y, Naitoh K, et al. In vivo effects by estrone sulfate on the central nervous system-senile dementia (Alzheimer's disease). J Steroid Biochem Mol Bio 1989;34:521.

46. Ohkura T, Isse K, Akazawa K, et al. Evaluation of estrogen treatment in female patients with dementia of the Alzheimer type. Endocr J 1994;41:361.

47. Ohkura T, Isse K, Akazawa K, et al. Low-dose estrogen replacement therapy for Alzheimer disease in women. Menopause 1994;1:125.

48. Honjo H, Ogino Y, Tanaka K, et al. An effect of conjugated estrogen to cognitive impariment in women with senile dementia—Alzheimer's type: a placebo-controlled double blind study. J Jpn Menopause Soc 1993;1:167.

49. Mulnard RA, Cotman CW, Koss E, et al. A multicenter, double-blind, placebo-controlled study of estrogen replacement therapy in patients with mild to moderate Alzheimer's disease: a pilot study of the Alzheimer's Disease Cooperative Research Unit (ADCSU). University of California at San Diego.

50. Women's Health Initiative, NIH. Bethesda, MD.

51. Schneider LS, Farlow MR, Henderson VW, et al. Effects of estrogen replacement therapy on response to tacrine in patients with Alzheimer's disease. Neurology 1996;46:1580.

CHAPTER 8

Movement Disorders

Michael Schwarzschild

Gender does not significantly influence the incidence of essential tremor, Parkinson's disease, or focal dystonias, which are the most common ailments seen in movement disorder clinics. However, a few uncommon movement disorders are unique to women or are disproportionately seen among them. This chapter reviews two such disorders: chorea gravidarum and chorea associated with systemic lupus erythematosus (SLE). The possible role of estrogen in these disorders as well as in Parkinson's disease and tardive dyskinesia is discussed.

Chorea Gravidarum

Chorea gravidarum is defined as involuntary, nonrhythmic jerky movements developing in pregnancy. Like many other descriptive diagnostic terms in neurology, chorea gravidarum generally presents a clear clinical picture that belies an underlying etiologic heterogeneity. Clinical and laboratory advances are yielding a better understanding of chorea gravidarum.

Until the 1980s, chorea gravidarum was considered a manifestation of Sydenham's (poststreptococcal) chorea presenting or recurring in pregnancy [1]. Since then, improved awareness and diagnosis of other causes of chorea during the reproductive years have modified this view. The appearance of chorea during pregnancy should prompt consideration of idiopathic autoimmune disorders (e.g., SLE) [2], neurodegenerative diseases such as Wilson's disease and Huntington's disease [3], coagulopathies and other causes of strokes, metabolic and endocrine disorders (e.g., hyperthyroidism), structural lesions, intoxications with illicit or prescription drugs (e.g., after stopping antiemetics or tapering neuroleptics), tardive movement disorders, and Sydenham's chorea [4]. The fact that many of these conditions are treatable underscores the importance of such a differential.

The incidence of chorea gravidarum has declined in large part because of the widespread use of effective antibiotic therapy for streptococcal infection. The roughly 40-fold drop in the incidence of chorea gravidarum from more than one in 4,000 pregnancies in the 1930s [4] to fewer than one in 100,000 pregnancies in the 1960s [5] reflects the effective prevention of Sydenham's chorea. Thus, the overall incidence of chorea during pregnancy has declined and the proportion of cases secondary to nonrheumatic etiologies has risen.

Natural History

Several characteristic clinical features of chorea gravidarum are common to the various etiologies, suggesting that hormonal changes during pregnancy, such as the relative elevated estrogen levels [6], may predispose a woman to the clinical expression of chorea. Chorea typically appears after the first month of pregnancy and may last for just a few days, but usually persists until delivery, with resolution over the following weeks. Recurrences are common in subsequent pregnancies [4]. Chorea is usually generalized but may be focal. Any strictly asymmetric presentation (i.e., true hemichorea) warrants careful assessment for a structural lesion or infarction.

Although symptoms were once considered highly dangerous to both mother and fetus, prompting the recommendation of therapeutic abortion by many as late as the 1960s [7], it is now clear that mortality and complications are comparable to those in normal pregnancies [8].

Evaluation

Appropriate assessment begins with a detailed history for previous rheumatic fever or chorea (Sydenham's), collagen-vascular disease symptoms, multiple spontaneous abortions or other clues to a hypercoagulable state, family history of movement disorder or psychiatric illness (e.g., autosomal recessive pattern in Wilson's disease and in some cases of chorea-acanthocytosis, and autosomal dominant pattern in Huntington's disease), and neuroleptic, antiemetic, anticonvulsant, or illicit drug use. Careful physical examination for associated systemic or neurologic signs includes evaluation for skin rash and other stigmata of collagen-vascular disease, aortic/mitral valve murmurs resulting from rheumatic fever, Kayser-Fleischer rings, and (particularly in cases of unilateral chorea) other focal neurologic deficits.

Laboratory evaluation may include serologic studies for SLE, such as antinuclear antibodies (ANA) or rheumatoid factor; a hypercoagulability screen (clotting times, anticardiolipin antibody/lupus anticoagulant, and, possibly, factor C, factor S, and antithrombin III levels); antistreptolysin titers and blood cultures for evidence of previous or active rheumatic fever; rapid plasma reagin to assess for cerebral syphilis; human immunodeficiency virus antibody; and serum ceruloplasmin and 24-hour urine copper levels as Wilson's disease markers. A peripheral blood smear showing more than 10% acanthocytes and an elevated serum creatine kinase level are suggestive of chorea-acanthocytosis. Hexosaminidase testing for Tay-Sachs may also be considered. An echocardiogram to look for signs of valvular disease may be warranted to pursue suspicion of rheumatic fever. If infarct, neoplasm, or focal infection are significant etiologic considerations, then the benefits of neuroimaging (preferably magnetic resonance imaging [MRI] without contrast agent during pregnancy) may outweigh any theoretic risk to the fetus. Otherwise, the MRI test may be deferred until the postpartum period. Neuroimaging may also support a diagnosis of Huntington's disease or Wilson's disease if structural changes in the basal ganglia such as caudate atrophy or neostriatal signal abnormalities, respectively, are found. Other causes of chorea gravidarum such as rheumatic fever [9] or antiphospholipid antibodies (lupus anticoagulant and anticardiolipin antibody) [10] have been associated with nonspecific MRI signal abnormalities.

Therapy

Treatment is best directed toward the underlying cause when it is identified. The wide differences between medical therapies for the treatable causes of chorea gravidarum highlight the importance of seeking a specific diagnosis. For example, a coagulopathy with circulating lupus anticoagulant in a woman with chorea gravidarum and progressive hemolysis has been successfully treated with prednisone and aspirin [10, 11], whereas Wilson's disease presenting with chorea gravidarum may be treated with copper chelation therapy.

As chorea gravidarum most commonly manifests with mild and self-limited chorea, symptomatic pharmacotherapy is usually not warranted. Minimizing the physical and psychological stresses that typically exacerbate chorea and avoiding situations in which sudden adventitious movements could prove harmful may be sufficient. Because all drugs useful in treating chorea have significant or unknown side effects on the developing fetus, they should be reserved for the unusual case in which the movements are so severe that maternal or fetal health is threatened. This may occur if incessant or violent movements lead to inadequate hydration or nutritional intake, rhabdomyolysis, hyperthermia, or insomnia. In such circumstances, haloperidol is the most widely recommended among the several medications tried for chorea gravidarum because of its proven efficacy and relatively low risk for the fetus [6]. Administration should be limited to the second and third trimesters given the inadequate data on teratogenicity, and total maternal exposure should be minimized to avoid complications such as tardive dyskinesia.

Chorea in Systemic Lupus Erythematosus

SLE is an autoimmune disorder involving multiple organs including the central and peripheral nervous system. Although up to 75% of patients develop neurologic symptoms, chorea occurs in less than 5% [12–16]. The pathogenesis of central nervous system (CNS) involvement in SLE remains unclear but may involve antibody deposition within the brain parenchyma, cerebral vasculitis, embolic lesions from cardiac valvular disease, and thromboses related to antiphospholipid antibodies—the latter most frequently implicated in lupus chorea [17]. In SLE the appearance of chorea is usually generalized but can be unilateral [18].

SLE with chorea occurs much more commonly in women, at least in part because of the gender differences in SLE incidence, with the disease almost 10 times more likely to be diagnosed in women than men. Given the diagnosis of SLE, it is controversial whether the risk of developing chorea is independent of gender. In some series the ratio of women to men is the same for SLE as it is for chorea in SLE [17]. However, chorea in SLE occurs more frequently in pregnancy, suggesting that cases of chorea gravidarum due to SLE increase the overall incidence of chorea in women with SLE [10].

The association with pregnancy again raises the possibility of a hormonal role in the development of chorea. Interestingly, oral contraceptives, which on their own have been implicated in the induction of chorea [19], may precipitate chorea as the initial presentation of SLE [20].

Appropriate treatment should focus on the underlying autoimmune disorder, reserving therapy with dopaminergic antagonists (e.g., haloperidol) for severe or unresponsive chorea [21]. The common treatment of CNS sequelae of SLE with corticosteroids remains controversial [22]. Although anti-inflammatory treatment has often been dramatically associated with resolution of symptoms, the chorea is often self-limiting and not always responsive to steroids. It should also be kept in mind that in the patient previously diagnosed with SLE and receiving immunosuppressive therapy, CNS infection must be considered with the development of any new neurologic symptom.

Course of Parkinson's Disease in Women

Although the incidence of Parkinson's disease is no greater in women than in men, its course can occasionally display features unique to women. Symptoms of Parkinson's disease in premenopausal women may fluctuate in synchrony with the menstrual cycle, with worsening during the week preceding menses [23, 24]. Moreover, pregnancy may have an exacerbating effect on parkinsonian symptoms [8, 25].

These and other data suggest that estrogens produce an antidopaminergic effect in Parkinson's disease [24]. A small double-blind crossover study of patients with Parkinson's disease found that three of four patients reported worsening parkinsonian symptoms with estrogen treatment but not with placebo [26]. Conversely, estrogen suppression with leuprolide was associated with improved parkinsonian symptoms in a 44-year-old woman with catamenial exacerbations [24]. Sound recommendations regarding estrogen use for postmenopausal women with Parkinson's disease cannot be made based on the largely anecdotal literature, and the topic is under more systematic study [27].

In contrast, the hyperkinetic movement disorder of tardive dyskinesia may be associated with relative hypoestrogenism, occurring with roughly twice the prevalence in postmenopausal women compared to men of the same age (whereas tardive dyskinesia in younger patients shows no gender specificity) [28, 29]. Thus a useful, if simplified, model emerges in which hypokinetic movement disorders such as Parkinson's disease may be exacerbated by higher levels of estrogen or related hormones and certain hyperkinetic movement disorders such as tardive dyskinesia may be facilitated by lower levels of these hormones.

References

1. Adams RD, Victor M. Principles of Neurology (3rd ed). New York: McGraw-Hill, 1985;61.
2. Donaldson IM, Espiner EA. Disseminated lupus erythematosus presenting as chorea gravidarum. Arch Neurol 1971;25:240.
3. Korenyi C, Whittier JR, Conchado D. Stress in Huntington's disease (chorea): review of the literature and personal observations. Dis Nerv Syst 1972;33:339.
4. Willson P, Preese AA. Chorea gravidarum. Arch Intern Med 1932;49:471.
5. Zegart KN, Schwarz RH. Chorea gravidarum. Obstet Gynecol 1968;32:24.
6. Donaldson JO. Control of chorea gravidarum with haloperidol. Obstet Gynecol 1982;59:381.
7. Lewis BV, Parsons M. Chorea gravidarum. Lancet 1966;1:284.
8. Golbe LI. Pregnancy and movement disorders. Neurologic complications of pregnancy. Neurol Clin 1994;12:497.
9. Ginnetti RA, Bredfeldt RC, Pegg EW. Chorea gravidarum: a case report including magnetic resonance imaging results. J Fam Pract 1989;29:87.
10. Omdal R, Roalsø S. Chorea gravidarum and chorea associated with oral contraceptives—diseases due to antiphospholipid antibodies? Acta Neurol Scand 1992;86:219.
11. Lubbe WF, Walker EB. Chorea gravidarum associated with circulating lupus anticoagulant: successful outcome of pregnancy with prednisone and aspirin therapy. Br J Obstet Gynaecol 1983;90:487.
12. Johnson RT, Richardson EP. The neurological manifestations of systemic lupus erythematosus. Medicine (Baltimore) 1968;47:337.
13. Bennhum DA, Messner RP. Recent observations on central nervous system lupus erythematosus. Semin Arthritis Rheum 1975;4:253.
14. Grigor R, Edmonds J, Lewkoonia R, et al. Systemic lupus erythematosus. A prospective analysis. Ann Rheum Dis 1978;37:121.

15. Sergent JS, Lockshin MD, Klempner MS, et al. Central nervous system disease in systemic lupus erythematosus. Am J Med 1975;58:644.

16. Feinglass EJ, Arnett FC, Dorsch CA, et al. Neuropsychiatric manifestations of systemic lupus erythematosus: diagnosis, clinical spectrum, and relationship to other features of the disease. Medicine 1976;55:323.

17. Asherson RA, Derksen RH, Harris EN, et al. Chorea in systemic lupus erythematosus and "lupus-like" disease: association with antiphospholipid antibodies. Semin Arthritis Rheum 1987;16:253.

18. Bruyn GW, Padberg G. Chorea and systemic lupus erythematosus: a critical review. Eur Neurol 1984;23:435.

19. Pulsinelli WA, Hamil RW. Chorea complicating oral contraceptive therapy: case report and review of the literature. Am J Med 1978;65:557.

20. Iskander MK, Khan MA. Chorea as the initial presentation of oral contraceptive related systemic lupus erythematosus. J Rheumatol 1989;16:850.

21. Agrawal BL, Foa RP. Collagen vascular disease appearing as chorea gravidarum. Arch Neurol 1982;39:192.

22. Wolf RE, McBeath JG. Chorea gravidarum in systemic lupus erythematosus. J Rheumatol 1985;12:992.

23. Quinn NP, Marsden CD. Menstrual-related fluctuations in Parkinson's disease. Mov Disord 1986;1:85.

24. Session DR, Pearlstone MM, Jewelewicz R, et al. Estrogens and Parkinson's disease. Med Hypoth 1994;42:280.

25. Golbe LI. Parkinson's disease and pregnancy. Neurology 1987;41:168.

26. Bédard P, Langelier P, Dankova J, et al. Estrogens, progesterone, and the extrapyramidal system. Adv Neurol 1979;24:411.

27. 1996 Clinical Studies at the National Institutes of Health, Clinical Center Communications. NIH Pub. No. 95-217. 1995;135.

28. Yassa R, Jeste DV. Gender differences in tardive dyskinesia: a critical review of the literature. Schizophr Bull 1992;18:701.

29. Muscettola G, Pampallona S, Barbato G, et al. Persistent tardive dyskinesia: demographic and pharmacological risk factors. Acta Psychiatr Scand 1993;87:29.

CHAPTER 9

Medical Conditions with Neurologic Manifestations

Alan Z. Segal

Medical illness in women frequently presents with prominent neurologic manifestations. Due to hormonal influences and other factors that are less well understood, Takayasu arteritis, systemic lupus erythematosus, thyroid disease, and the other conditions discussed here occur more often in women [1]. Neurologic signs may present at disease onset or appear as a primary manifestation of established disease, making the neurologic evaluation central to diagnosis and treatment.

Takayasu Arteritis

Takayasu arteritis (TA), or pulseless disease, is a chronic, idiopathic, inflammatory disease that primarily affects large vessels such as the aorta and its main branches. The illness was first described in Asia but is now more frequently recognized in Western Europe and North America. In the United States, the estimated incidence is 2.6 cases per million per year. The most comprehensive series to date, compiled by the National Institutes of Health (NIH), included 60 patients who were almost exclusively women of reproductive age (97%). The etiology of this overwhelming predominance is not known. Whites comprised a majority at 75%. Although Asians comprised only 10%, this figure was in excess of a 2.9% representation in the general population. This ethnic predilection has raised questions about the possible predisposing role of human leukocyte antigens (HLAs). Of Japanese patients with TA, 50% have association with Bw52 and DR12 antigens when compared with healthy controls, while American patients show a predominance of the DR4 and MB3 antigens. The median

139

age of onset of TA in this study was 25 years, with 35% of patients presenting in the third decade and 32% presenting before age 20 [2]. Strictly defined, TA must occur before age 40 [3], but clinically convincing cases often occur beyond that age.

The etiology of TA is unknown. Infections with spirochetes, tuberculosis, or streptococcus have been postulated as the origin, but this has not been supported with further evidence. An autoimmune cause with pathogenic antiaortic antibodies has also been postulated. Pathologically, there is a granulomatous panarteritis. Endothelial proliferation leads to intimal thickening, fibrosis, and luminal narrowing.

The classic clinical course of TA is triphasic, characterized by prepulseless inflammation followed by a painful ischemic period and finally ending in burned-out, fibrotic pulseless disease. Vascular findings are necessary for the diagnosis of TA, but these stages are not invariable. Arteries typically become tender and extremities (particularly the arms) cool, and claudication occurs [4]. In the NIH series, 80% of the 60 patients had a bruit, mostly commonly carotid (70%), with a high rate of carotidynia (32%). Multiple bruits were found in 33% of patients, with an upper extremity predominance. Lesions tended to be stenotic and less frequently formed aneurysms. Hypertension was present in 33% of patients and was usually independent of renal artery stenosis, which occurred in only 2% [2].

Systemic constitutional symptoms such as fatigue, malaise, myalgias, arthralgias, fever, and weight loss are not only nonspecific for TA but manifested in a minority of the NIH patients, with only 33% seen on presentation and 43% at any time during the disease course. Other cohorts, however, did show a higher rate of systemic signs, with arthralgia and arthritis or myalgia noted in the majority of patients [5]. Skin manifestations such as erythema nodosum are rare and nonspecific. Biopsy of skin is unhelpful.

Neurologic symptoms are common. Lightheadedness and dizziness occurred in one-third of patients in the NIH series and correlated with vertebral artery (VA) stenosis. It was found that 57% of patients with VA stenosis were lightheaded, compared with 23% of those without it. It is not clear what portion of these patients had evidence of brain stem vestibular dysfunction due to focal ischemia as compared to more global hypoperfusion with lightheadedness. Since the majority of VA stenoses (>80%) were unilateral, the former is more likely. Headache was common (42%) but was not associated with carotid or vertebral disease.

Visual disturbances, in most cases binocular blurring, occurred in 48% of patients with VA involvement as compared to 18% of patients without. Visual complaints also correlated with carotid disease, which was seen in 40% of patients with carotid disease and 12% of patients without. Most carotid stenoses were bilateral. There was one case of transient monocular blindness [2].

Ten of the 60 patients had transient ischemic attacks or strokes, the majority with lesions that correlated with a site of stenosis, the others occurring secondary to hypertension. Two of these patients had residual hemiparesis and one had persistent monocular blindness [2].

Patterns of perfusion in TA may be complex. Even in the absence of discrete carotid or vertebral disease, there may be reversal of flow in the vertebral arteries with subclavian steal. Alternatively, decreased flow in the aortic arch may directly reduce anterior/posterior circulation flow leading to borderline ischemia [6]. Finally, the integrity of the circle of Willis and intracranial vessels may not be normal, with intrinsic disease in these vessels limiting collateral circulation. Involvement of the major intracranial arteries (anterior, middle, and posterior) occurs, often as an extension of internal carotid or basilar disease. Due to the variability of flow patterns, the extent of stenosis on angiogram may not provide sufficient evidence of end-organ hypoperfusion [7]. Doppler ultrasound, single photon emission computed tomography, positron emission tomography, computed tomography (CT) angiography or magnetic resonance (MR) with perfusion imaging, MR angiography, or MR cine protocols might allow better differentiation of territory at risk [8].

Other laboratory tests are of limited value. The sedimentation rate is elevated in 72% of patients with active disease but is not sufficiently sensitive. Of the four patients in the NIH series with positive biopsies for vasculitis, only one had an elevated erythrocyte sedimentation rate. Other laboratory findings such as anemia, thrombocytosis, leukocytosis, and hypergammaglobulinemia occur but are nonspecific. Chest radiographs may show widening of the mediastinum. Arteriography, as noted above, is the standard means of diagnosis but cannot differentiate between acute and chronic lesions. Biopsy material of a large-sized artery is preferable, but given the obvious risks involved, such tissue is usually obtained only at the time of bypass surgery.

Unlike collagen vascular disease in general, TA is for the most part unaffected by pregnancy, and successful childbirth is not uncommon. In the NIH series, five patients became pregnant, all had normal spontaneous vaginal deliveries, and only one had exacerbation of TA. Other published reports also confirm good maternal and fetal outcomes [9]. Some even show a possible beneficial effect of pregnancy, perhaps due to vasodilatory effects of circulating prostaglandins, with increased pulse amplitude demonstrated on digital plethysmography [10].

Treatment is best initiated during the acute, inflammatory, prepulseless phase, during which damage may be reversible. Early diagnosis is therefore crucial. TA is very responsive to steroids, which produce a 60% remission rate when used alone. Cytotoxic agents can be used if steroids have failed or to avoid the use of steroids. Methotrexate is the best-established treatment; however, azathioprine and cyclophosphamide have also been used with success [7].

Surgical treatment is indicated if uncontrolled hypertension requires renal artery bypass, extremity ischemia limits activities of daily living, or carotid stenosis is greater than 70%. It is unlikely that the large clinical trials of carotid endarterectomy such as the North American Symptomatic Carotid Endarterectomy Trial could be extrapolated to TA cases. Surgery is also indicated for aortic insufficiency (grade 2 or worse), which can also be a limiting factor in central nervous system (CNS) perfusion. Finally, coronary artery disease may require bypass surgery. Ischemia-related arrhythmias may also produce neurologic complications if periods of generalized hypoperfusion occur.

In the NIH series, bypass grafts were performed in nine of 60 patients for symptomatic carotid stenosis. These were performed with the ascending aorta as the proximal anastomotic site. Bypass with Dacron or saphenous vein graft, rather than endarterectomy, minimizes but does not eliminate the possibility of TA recurrence at the surgical site. Nineteen patients had subcritical stenoses or stenoses in distributions that could not be bypassed safely [2].

Systemic Lupus Erythematosus

Systemic lupus erythematosus (SLE) is a disease of unknown etiology in which multiple organ systems are damaged by circulating autoantibodies and immune complexes. Over 80% of SLE patients are women. While the female-to-male ratio in children is only 1.4 to 1.0, this ratio increases to 8 to 1 in patients of childbearing age (ages 20–39) and decreases to 5 to 1 in the population aged 40–64 and 2 to 1 in older patients [4]. Mouse models of the disease as well as its clinical course indicate a prominent hormone-mediated effect. Both endogenous and exogenous estrogens as well as decreased androgen concentrations have been reported to worsen SLE. Menopausal patients on hormone replacement therapy with estrogen have a doubled relative risk of SLE [11], and patients taking oral contraceptives have an increase in SLE flares [12]. Other studies, however, dispute these relationships [13].

The profound female predominance seen in SLE is common with a number of other collagen vascular diseases, including Sjögren's syndrome, rheumatoid arthritis, and scleroderma (discussed later in this chapter). This predominance does not apply to all rheumatologic disease, however. For unknown reasons, Reiter's syndrome and ankylosing spondylitis are more common in men [14].

Neurologic manifestations can be the presenting complaint for SLE patients or may occur in the setting of established disease. Although the American Rheumatologic Association definition of CNS SLE includes only seizures and psychosis, neurologic manifestations vary far more widely. As shown in Table 9.1, neuropsychiatric SLE (NPSLE) can be generally classi-

TABLE 9.1
Neuropsychiatric Manifestations in Systemic Lupus Erythematosus

Central nervous system
Diffuse manifestations (35–60%)
   Organic brain syndromes
      Organic amnestic/cognitive dysfunction
      Dementia
      Altered consciousness
   Psychiatric
      Psychosis
      Organic mood/anxiety syndromes
Seizures (15–35%)
   Grand mal
   Focal
   Petit mal
   Temporal lobe
Focal manifestations
   Cranial neuropathies
   Cerebrovascular accidents/strokes
   Transverse myelitis
   Movement disorders
Other
   Headaches
   Aseptic meningitis
   Pseudotumor cerebri
   Normal pressure hydrocephalus

Peripheral nervous system
Peripheral neuropathies (10–20%)
   Sensory polyneuropathy
   Mononeuritis multiplex
   Chronic, relapsing polyneuropathy
   Guillain-Barré syndrome
Other
   Autonomic neuropathy
   Myasthenia gravis
   Eaton-Lambert syndrome

fied into global (diffuse) and focal (with discrete strokelike events), a division that correlates with presumed pathophysiology.

Focal events probably relate to the presence of antiphospholipid (aPL) antibodies (see Chapter 2). Vascular occlusion occurs on a thrombotic basis and can affect either large or small vessels. On biopsy, vascular changes are not prominently vasculitic. Instead, a bland vasculopathy occurs with endothelial proliferation and fibrosis. These lesions may represent the terminal phases of a healed or treated vasculitic process or may be related to the binding of aPL antibodies to endothelial cells and platelets. Embolic events can also occur as a result of cardiac valvular vegetations in Libman-Sacks endocarditis [15]. The thrombotic and embolic complications of aPL antibodies are discussed further in Chapter 2.

Global effects on the brain may be mediated by a number of brain-reactive antibodies including antineuronal, antiribosomal P, antiastrocyte, antineurofilament, and anti-MAG or anti-GM_1 antibodies. The target antigen of antineuronal antibodies has been shown to be an integral 50-kd membrane protein isolated by Western blot and enzyme-linked immunosorbent assays using in vitro preparations of axonal and synaptic membranes [16]. These antibodies cross-react with brain tissue and circulating lymphocytes [17]. Experimental injection of these antibodies into cortical tissue or ventricles leads to meningitis, seizures, and motor dysfunction in animals [4].

The precise pathogenesis of these antibodies in humans is unclear. They are nonspecific, present both in non–CNS SLE patients and in patients with other inflammatory states without CNS involvement. Antibodies may be a byproduct of an inflammatory state rather than the direct mechanism of injury. Furthermore, for antibodies to be pathogenic, passage through the blood-brain barrier or in situ CNS production would be required. Cerebrospinal fluid (CSF) measurement of antibodies can be performed but does not add to sensitivity or specificity. Some studies have shown high correlations between serum antineuronal antibodies and cognitive impairment with titer fluctuations varying with clinical flares. However, others have failed to confirm this relationship. In one study, neuropsychiatric manifestations were seen in 60% of SLE patients who had antineuronal antibodies, compared to 7–12% of patients with aPL antibodies. Among SLE patients, antineuronal antibodies were seen in 32% of patients with CNS SLE but also in 23% of those without [16]. Patients with seizures related to SLE also have high antibody titers, but these are also seen in patients with seizure disorders unrelated to SLE and may be a byproduct rather than the cause of seizure activity [18].

A more reliable correlation exists for antiribosomal P antibodies, particularly in psychiatric disease. Bonfa found these antibodies in 90% of SLE patients with psychosis, compared to 12% of patients without psychosis [19]. Schneebaum showed antiribosomal P in 88% of patients with depression, compared to 45% with psychosis and only 9% in patients with no psychiatric disease [20].

Antiastrocyte (vimentin) and antineurofilament antibodies have also been measured and do not correlate with disease activity [16]. Anti-MAG antibodies, which are associated with peripheral nervous system and CNS demyelination, are increased in SLE patients [21]. Anti-GM_1 antibodies reactive against brain tissue antigens have also been documented in SLE patients [22].

Diffuse presentations of NPSLE include prominent cognitive and behavioral changes. The most frequent change seen is depression, often accompanied by mild subjective cognitive complaints. The depression most closely correlates with SLE disease activity when accompanied by organic manifestations such as visual hallucinations or poorly organized delusions. A prominent feature of the depression, however, may be reactive rather than primary and may be a side effect of disease treatment with corticosteroids. Although psychosis occurs in up to 15% of patients with CNS SLE, a majority of these cases may be steroid induced. Anxiety and manic symptoms have also been described. Nonspecific confusion and decreased alertness can occur, often in the setting of concurrent medical complications. Memory can be affected acutely or chronic dementia can occur. Dementia may be a manifestation of persistently active NPSLE, scarring from previously active disease, or in the setting of multiple infarcts from anticardiolipin (aCL) antibodies. Stupor and coma occur in a small minority. There is increased mortality rate with SLE if there are neuropsychiatric manifestations. NPSLE may not, however, be the cause but merely a marker for severe disease overall, often occurring in the setting of infection, renal failure, and severe disability [15, 23].

Seizures are frequent in CNS SLE, occurring in one-third of patients in some series. These may be generalized, simple, or complex-partial with electroencephalogram (EEG) changes correlating with seizure type and location. Multiple factors in addition to SLE itself contribute to seizures in these cases, including underlying infection, azotemia, or focal stroke. Seizure frequency correlates with severity of flares [18].

Migraine headaches are increased in SLE and may occur in the setting of aPL antibodies. Pseudotumor cerebri may develop as a result of dural venous sinus thrombosis, with or without aPL antibodies, or as a result of rapid steroid withdrawal. Other forms of headache, such as tension or muscle contraction pain, are also more common in SLE [4, 15].

Focal demyelination leading to cerebral white matter disease or transverse myelitis may occur and may be difficult to distinguish from multiple sclerosis (MS). The term *lupoid sclerosis* has been applied. These patients' clinical presentation closely resembles MS, but they have laboratory findings suggestive of SLE, including ANA (titer usually >1:1,000), false-positive tests for syphilis, and aPL antibodies. Other investigators have found anti-MAG antibodies, a possible sign of direct antibody-mediated myelin damage. Antimyelin antibodies have also been seen in MS but are not thought to be the pathogenesis of that disease [24].

Ataxia, parkinsonian rigidity or tremor, hemiballismus, and, most commonly, chorea occur, often in the absence of documentable lesions in the cerebellum or basal ganglia [25]. Only two of 10 cases of SLE-related chorea had basal ganglia lesions at autopsy. SLE-related chorea is clinically similar to Sydenham's chorea from rheumatic fever and the two conditions may be linked by a common antineuronal antibody. However, SLE-related chorea has also been associated with an increased frequency of aPL antibodies [18].

Peripheral nerve manifestations can occur on a vasculitic basis, with focal infarction of the vasa nervorum. This may manifest initially as a mononeuritis multiplex and then evolve into a distal polyneuropathy [15]. Clinically, this polyneuropathy is diffuse, often with prominent decreased vibration sense and demyelinating features on electromyography—21% show decreased nerve conduction velocity, compared to 6% in controls [26]. Autonomic neuropathy has also been shown to occur, manifesting as decreased cardiac response to orthostasis [27]. Also, cranial neuropathies affecting the cranial nerves III and VI, Bell's palsy, trigeminal neuralgia, or optic neuropathy can occur. Optic neuropathy may be ischemic (in the setting of aPL antibodies) or demyelinating [15]. Guillain-Barré syndrome and chronic inflammatory demyelinating polyneuropathy have been reported [28].

Presence of a CSF inflammatory state is variable. Only 20–50% of patients have elevated protein and 6–34% have pleocytosis [15, 29]. Oligoclonal bands (OCBs) were seen in 25% of patients with NPSLE. CSF inflammation, (i.e., positive OCBs and an elevated IgG-to-albumin ratio) correlates closely with diffuse but not focal presentations of NPSLE. Clinically apparent aseptic meningitis occurs rarely. Patients with psychiatric manifestations may show ventricular enlargement, widened cortical sulci and calcifications on CT, or multifocal T2 hyperintensities on MRI, but findings are usually normal [30].

Treatment of the neurologic complications of SLE must be tailored to the individual situation. Steroids, either oral prednisone at doses of 1 mg/kg per day or high-dose pulse steroids, at an approximate IV dose of 1 g methylprednisolone, can be considered. In patients who present with psychiatric symptoms during steroid treatment, in whom a SLE flare cannot be differentiated from steroid psychosis, steroids may be transiently increased empirically, then tapered rapidly if no improvement or worsening occurs. Steroids should also be avoided in patients with cognitive complaints that may be chronic or may have a nonorganic basis. Other immune modulators such as cyclophosphamide, plasmapheresis, or intravenous immunoglobulin may be used in certain cases, but their use has not been systematically studied.

The effect of pregnancy on SLE is minimal, but its precise effect is controversial. While large-scale studies show that pregnancy does not cause a significant increase in SLE manifestations, other series show that as many as 74% of SLE patients experience a flare during pregnancy or during the 6 weeks postpartum. It is unclear whether worsening of SLE during pregnancy is due to pregnancy itself or due to the withdrawal of immune suppressants such as azathioprine or steroids, which may be contraindicated during pregnancy.

Fertility rates are normal in SLE patients, but spontaneous abortion and stillbirth are common, especially with the presence of aPL antibodies;

either aCL, IgG, or IgM; or lupus anticoagulant. In one series of SLE patients in which aPL status was not known, the rate of stillbirths was 24%, with 33% preterm deliveries and 33% with fetal growth retardation [31]. In patients with known aPL antibodies, fetal loss rates were over 50%. Fetal outcome also closely correlates with maternal renal disease, particularly persistent proteinuria. Fetal outcome can be further compromised by neonatal lupus, mediated by transplacental passage of IgG anti–SS-A (Ro) and anti–SS-B (La) from the mother. The syndrome is transient and relatively uncommon, seen in 4% of infants born to mothers with SLE. Heart block occurs in a small portion of these and is caused by inflammation or fibrosis in the either the atrioventricular node, bundle of His, or both. Heart block may lead to Stokes-Adams attacks, but is often asymptomatic [32]. Treatment for women with a history of fetal loss and aCL antibodies is aspirin. High-dose steroids, subcutaneous heparin, or warfarin (Coumadin) in full anticoagulating doses may be considered. If contraception is desired, use of progesterone preparations alone or low-dose estrogens is preferable [4].

Sjögren's Syndrome

Sjögren's syndrome is an immunologic disorder marked by exocrine glandular inflammation leading to sicca complex and varied other autoimmune phenomena. Sjögren's syndrome has a 9-to-1 female-to-male predominance and is probably not related to estrogen stimulation. Rather, the disease may be triggered by estrogen deprivation. It tends to flare at the onset of menopause, and in contrast to SLE, hormone replacement therapy has no effect on the disease [33].

Neurologic compromise can occur in primary Sjögren's syndrome or in association with other connective tissue diseases in its secondary form [12]. Neurologic complications occur in approximately 20–70% with a wide variation between series [34]. Peripheral neuropathy occurs frequently and can be the presenting manifestation in the setting of previously unrecognized sicca complex [35]. Distal nerves are most often affected, manifesting as a symmetric sensory polyneuropathy. Dorsal root ganglia and proximal nerves can also be affected. Large fibers are preferentially damaged, leading to an ataxic sensory neuropathy resembling tabes dorsalis. Autonomic neuropathy, manifested as Adie's pupil, or fixed tachycardia with orthostatic hypotension, is also common. The neuropathy may be demyelinating but is usually destructive and axonal, related to vasculitic involvement of the endoneurium [36]. Mononeuropathies are relatively rare in Sjögren's syndrome compared to other collagen vascular diseases, but isolated cranial neuropathies, especially trigeminal neuropathy, occur commonly.

Primary Sjögren's syndrome can also present with multifocal, recurrent, and progressive CNS disease such as hemiparesis, transverse myelopathy, hemisensory defects, seizures, and movement disorders. CNS Sjögren's syndrome often mimics MS and may only be differentiated by the addition of sicca complex or a positive minor salivary gland biopsy. The presence of vasculitis documented on skin biopsy may also distinguish primary Sjögren's syndrome from MS. Generalized cognitive dysfunction and depression occur frequently, as in NPSLE. CSF usually shows a lymphocytic pleocytosis, with OCBs similar to those seen in MS. Optic neuritis is common, seen in over half the patients in one series [36]. CNS Sjögren's syndrome, NPSLE, and MS likely exist on a continuum, differentiated less by their neurologic findings than by serologic tests and concomitant connective tissue disease manifestations. Diagnosis is crucial because the dementia-like picture caused by these entities may be reversible with corticosteroid therapy [38].

Rheumatoid Arthritis

Rheumatoid arthritis (RA), a multisystem disease most prominently causing a polyarthritis, affects women three times more often than men. As in Sjögren's syndrome, the etiology of this predominance may not be hormonal. RA tends to improve during pregnancy (at a time of elevated estrogen levels), perhaps due to changes in T-cell regulation [39]. Neurologic impairment can occur when a vasculitic component is present, causing a polyneuropathy closely resembling that of Sjögren's syndrome. More frequent, however, are local, mechanical compressive complications. Mononeuropathies occur due to nerves entrapped by proliferative synovitis or joint deformities, most frequently at median, ulnar, radial, or anterior tibial nerves.

Myelopathy due to atlantoaxial subluxation is a major concern. Disease of the synovial lining leads to ligamentous laxity, particularly in the transverse ligament. The skull and atlas are displaced forward on the axis, with relative backward movement of the odontoid. Pain radiating up to the occiput in a C2 distribution is common, and a slowly progressive spastic quadriparesis evolves with painless sensory loss and atrophy in the hands. Root pain in the arms is less frequent and serves to differentiate RA spondyloarthropathy from cervical spine disease at lower levels. Multiple partial subluxations of C2–C6 leads to the condition termed *staircase spine*.

Pathologic data show that cord compromise at C1–C2 is not directly due to mechanical contusion of the cord, but rather as a result of vascular compromise of the anterior spinal artery and venous system. The degree of subluxation may be less of a determinant of risk than underlying individual anatomic variation in the diameter of the spinal canal. Transient episodes of medullary and pontine dysfunction characterized by nystagmus, diplopia, and slurred speech also occur. This may be due to direct vertebral penetration of the dens into the medulla but, again, is more likely a result of vertebral artery compromise [40]. A high index of suspicion for spinal cord compromise is needed, since diagnosis in this population can be difficult because of superimposed periarticular muscle atrophy, compressive neuropathies, and joint deformities [4].

During childbirth, patients with RA may be at a high risk for cervical cord compression. Joint laxity increases during pregnancy and is compounded by the added mechanical stress of childbearing. Care should be paid to the cervical spine during labor if there is a history of underlying subluxation [32].

Scleroderma

Progressive systemic sclerosis (PSS), or scleroderma, affects women three times more often than men, with an even higher ratio during childbearing years [41]. Estrogen may play a part in etiology, as 40% of cases flare during pregnancy [38]. Although neurologic disease is not classically considered as a complication of PSS, a recent cohort noted neurologic manifestations in 40% of patients. Myopathy was the most frequent, occurring in 22% of patients. This myopathy can vary between a simple myopathy, polymyositis, or, rarely, inclusion body myositis. Peripheral neuropathy also occurs, as in RA, particularly when vasculitis is associated with PSS. The mechanism of injury is primarily microangiopathic due to vasculitis (as in SLE or Sjögren's syndrome), but fibrotic nerve entrapment, which is more similar to RA, can occur. Myelopathy has also been observed with predominantly posterolateral column dysfunction; however, no clear etiology has been offered. Cerebrovascular complications occur rarely. CSF protein is mildly increased. Metabolic derangements, especially vitamin deficiencies, should be considered in patients with neurologic disease and prominent gastrointestinal tract dysfunction. Although measurable parameters have not been found abnormal in these patients, malabsorption of an unknown factor remains possible [42].

Thyroid Disease

Autoimmune thyroid disease, including Graves' and Hashimoto's diseases, occurs predominantly in women. Because of this, hyperthyroidism is five times more frequent in women than men and hypothyroidism is ten times more common in women [43]. Unlike the collagen vascular diseases, it is unlikely that sex steroids play a role in this relationship.

The neurologic presentation of hyperthyroidism includes nervousness, emotional lability, and hyperkinesia. Tremor of the hands, tongue, or eyelids may mimic parkinsonism or worsen a pre-existing parkinsonian tremor. Chorea and paroxysmal athetosis can occur, probably due to sympathetic overactivity and catecholamine excess. Frequency of seizures may increase in a patient with known convulsions. EEG may show triphasic waves, which resolve with treatment of the hyperthyroidism.

There is a significant concordance between Graves' disease and myasthenia gravis (MG). Graves' disease occurs in 3–5% of patients with MG, and 1% of Graves' disease patients also have MG. The combination of ptosis, diplopia, and proximal muscle weakness due to myasthenia may be partly related to concomitant Graves' disease.

Ocular complications of Graves' disease may be due to either spastic or mechanical causes. In the former, sympathetic overactivity affects Müller's muscle in the upper eyelids and creates a widened palpebral fissure. There is infrequent blink rate and lid lag. Mechanically, orbital edema and infiltration by inflammatory cells leads to orbital fullness, conjunctival edema, hyperemia, and proptosis. Optic neuropathy may occur due to compression or ischemia, with decreased blood supply from high intraocular pressures. Graves' ophthalmopathy, if unilateral, should raise concern of orbital neoplasms, carotid-cavernous fistula, cavernous sinus thrombosis, or infiltrative disorders of the orbit.

Hyperthyroid myopathy causes proximal muscle weakness, most prominently in the legs. Presentation is nonspecific and can precede the diagnosis of hyperthyroidism. The severity of myopathy does not correlate with levels of thyroid hormone. In contrast to the proximal weakness of chronic hyperthyroidism, acute thyroid hormone excess leads to a toxic myopathy that is distal and often affects bulbar muscles. Corticospinal tract involvement due to hyperthyroidism can also occur, but is a diagnosis of exclusion after more common causes are ruled out.

Thyrotoxic periodic paralysis can occur and is characterized by episodic attacks of profound weakness precipitated by a large carbohydrate load or strenuous exercise. Hypokalemia occurs due to a combination of insulin release and sympathetic activity with beta-adrenergic stimulation causing passage of potassium into cells.

Hypothyroidism presents most frequently with mental status change including apathy and poor concentration progressing to confusion and psychosis (myxedema madness–coma). Myopathy is common. Muscle discomfort is greater at night and is exacerbated by prolonged, repetitive activity. Slowed relaxation of reflexes may be the only objective finding. Hoffman's atrophy with weakness but increased muscle mass and pseudohypertrophy also occurs. Sensorineural hearing loss has been attributed to temporal bone hypertrophy but studies have failed to document morphologic changes in the bone. Both mononeuropathy and polyneuropathy have been described. The former may be due to compression by connective tissue accumulation in the nerve sheath and most commonly occurs at the median nerve. Sensory polyneuropathies are usually small fiber and can be painful. Thyroid enlargement in Hashimoto's disease can compress the recurrent laryngeal nerve or the sympathetic chain, leading to Horner's syndrome [44].

Prolactinoma

Prolactinomas are the most commonly occurring pituitary tumor. Microadenomas occur more frequently in women (90%), while 60% of macroadenomas are found in men. Because these tumors create endocrine symptoms such as irregular menses, amenorrhea, and galactorrhea, they are detected at an earlier, often microscopic, phase in females. However, a more aggressive tumor biology in men, as opposed to insidious growth, has not been excluded. As prolactinomas enlarge, headaches or visual disturbances, most classically a bitemporal hemianopia, occur. Pregnancy may lead to tumor enlargement in approximately 15% of patients, usually during the first trimester. In addition to prolactin, pituitary adenomas frequently secrete growth hormone or adrenocorticotropic hormone and produce Cushing's syndrome, a possible cause of unexplained hypertension in a young woman [41].

References

1. Beeson PB. Age and sex associations of 40 autoimmune diseases. Am J Med 1994;96:457.
2. Kerr GS, Hallahan CW, Giordano J, et al. Takayasu arteritis. Ann Intern Med 1994;120:919.
3. Sharma BK, Siveski-Iliskovic N, Singal PK. Takayasu arteritis may be underdiagnosed in North America. Can J Cardiol 1995;11:311.
4. Conn DL, Hunder GG, O'Duffy JD. Vasculitis and Related Disorders. In WN Kelley, ED Harris, S Ruddy, et al. (eds), Textbook of Rheumatology. Philadelphia: Saunders, 1993;1077.
5. Hall S, Barr W, Lie JT, et al. Takayasu arteritis. Medicine 1985;64:89.
6. Grosset DG, Patterson J, Bone I. Intracranial haemodynamics in Takayasu's arteritis. Acta Neurochir 1992;119:161.
7. Kerr GS. Takayasu's arteritis. Curr Opin Rheumatol 1994;6:32.
8. Takano K, Sadoshima S, Ibayashi S, et al. Altered cerebral hemodynamics and metabolism in Takayasu arteritis with neurologic deficits. Stroke 1993;24:1501.
9. Bassa A, Desai DK, Moodley J. Takayasu's disease and pregnancy. Three case studies and a review of the literature. S Afr Med J 1995;85:107.
10. Matsumura A, Moriwaki R, Numano F. Pregnancy in Takayasu arteritis from the view of internal medicine. Heart Vessels Suppl 1992;7:120.
11. Sanchez-Guerrero J, Liang MH, Karlson EW. Postmenopausal estrogen therapy and the risk for developing systemic lupus erythematosus. Ann Intern Med 1995;122:430.
12. McCarty DJ, Koopman WJ. Arthritis and Allied Conditions. Philadelphia: Lea & Febiger, 1993;1156.
13. Boumpas DT, Fessler BJ, Austin HA III, et al. Systemic lupus erythematosus: emerging concepts. Part 2: Dermatologic and joint disease, the antiphospho-

lipid antibody syndrome, pregnancy and hormonal therapy, morbidity and mortality, and pathogenesis. Ann Intern Med 1995;123:42.

14. Atkinson, JP. Some thoughts on autoimmunity. Arthritis Rheum 1995;38:301.
15. West SG. Neuropsychiatric lupus. Rheum Dis Clin North Am 1994;20:129.
16. Hay EM, Isenberg DA. Autoantibodies in central nervous system lupus. Br J Rheumatol 1993;32:329.
17. Denburg JA, Behmann SA. Lymphocyte and neuronal antigens in neuropsychiatric lupus: presence of an elutable, immunoprecipitable lymphocyte/neuronal 52 kd reactivity. Ann Rheum Dis 1994;53:304.
18. Futrell N, Schultz LR, Millikan C. Central nervous system disease in patients with systemic lupus erythematosus. Neurology 1992;42:1649.
19. Bonfa E, Golombek SJ, Kaufman LD, et al. Association between lupus psychosis and antiribosomal-P protein antibodies. N Engl J Med 1987;317:265.
20. Schneebaum AB, Singleton JD, West SG, et al. Association of psychiatric manifestations with antibodies to ribosomal P proteins in systemic lupus erythematosus. Am J Med 1991;90:54.
21. Khalili A, Cooper RC. A study of immune response to myelin and cardiolipin in patients with systemic lupus erythematosus. Clin Exp Immunol 1991;85:365.
22. Hirano T, Hashimoto H, Shiokawa Y. Autoantibodies in central nervous system lupus. Br J Rheum 1993;32:329.
23. Miguel EC, Pereira RM, Pereira CA. Psychiatric manifestations of systemic lupus erythematosus: clinical features, symptoms, and signs of central nervous system activity in 43 patients. Medicine 1994;73:224.
24. Marullo S, Clauvel J-P, Intrator L, et al. Lupoid sclerosis with antiphospholipid and antimyelin antibodies. J Rheumatol 1993;20:747.
25. Vidakovic A, Dragasevic N, Kostic VS. Hemiballism: report of 25 cases. J Neurol Neurosurg Psychiatry 1994;57:945.
26. Omdal R, Mellgren SI, Husby G. A controlled study of peripheral neuropathy in systemic lupus erythematosus. Acta Neurol Scand 1993;88:41.
27. Liote F, Osterland CK. Autonomic neuropathy in systemic lupus erythematosus: cardiovascular autonomic function assessment. Ann Rheum Dis 1994;53:671.
28. Robson MG, Walport MJ, Davies KA. Systemic lupus erythematosus and acute demyelinating polyneuropathy. Br J Rheumatol 1994;33:1074.
29. McLean BN, Miller D, Thomson EJ. Oligoclonal banding of IgG in CSF, blood-brain barrier function, and MRI findings in patients with sarcoidosis, systemic lupus erythematosus, and Behçet's disease involving the nervous system. J Neurol Neurosurg Psychiatry 1995;58:548.
30. West SG, Emlen W, Wener MH, et al. Neuropsychiatric lupus erythematosus: a 10-year prospective study on the value of diagnostic tests. Am J Med 1995;99:153.
31. Fine LG, Barnett EV, Danovitch GM, et al. Systemic lupus erythematosus in pregnancy. Ann Intern Med 1981;94:667.

32. Cunningham FG, McDonald PC. Obstetrics. Norwalk, CT: Appleton & Lange, 1993.
33. Lehrer S, Bogursky E, Yemini M, et al. Gynecologic manifestations of Sjögren's syndrome. Am J Obstet Gynecol 1994;170:835.
34. Volk ME, Kratzsch G, Krapf H, et al. Neurologic and neuropsychiatric dysfunction in primary Sjögren's syndrome. Acta Neurol Scand 1994;89:31.
35. Gemignani F, Marbini A, Pavesi G, et al. Peripheral neuropathy associated with primary Sjögren's syndrome. J Neurol Neurosurg Psychiatry 1994;57:983.
36. Griffin, Cornblath DR, Alexander E, et al. Ataxic sensory neuropathy and dorsal root ganglionitis associated with Sjögren's syndrome. Ann Neurol 1990;27:304.
37. Alexander EL, Malinow K, Lejewski BS, et al. Primary Sjögren's syndrome with central nervous disease mimicking multiple sclerosis. Ann Intern Med 1986;104:323.
38. Casselli RJ, Scheithauer BW, Bowles CA, et al. The treatable dementia of Sjögren's syndrome. Ann Neurol 1991;30:98.
39. Buyon JP, Yaron M, Lockshin MD. First international conference on rheumatologic disease in pregnancy. Arthritis Rheum 1993;36:59.
40. Nakano KK, Schoene WC, Baker RA, et al. The cervical myelopathy associated with rheumatoid arthritis: analysis of 32 patients, with 2 postmortem cases. Ann Neurol 1978;3:144.
41. Gilliland BC. Systemic Sclerosis. In KJ Isselbacher, E Braunwald (eds), Principles of Internal Medicine. New York: McGraw-Hill, 1994;1655.
42. Averbuch-Heller L, Steiner I, Abramsky O. Neurologic manifestations of progressive systemic sclerosis. Arch Neurol 1992;49:1292.
43. Benjamin F. Endocrine Disorders. In VL Seltzer, WH Pearse (eds), Women's Primary Health Care. New York: McGraw-Hill, 1995;525.
44. Tonner DR, Schlechte JA. Neurologic complications of thyroid and parathyroid disease. Med Clin North Am 1993;77:251.

Index